THE COMPLETE GUIDE TO SURF FITNESS

DEDICATED TO THE MEMORY OF MIKE PHELPS
1933 - 2009

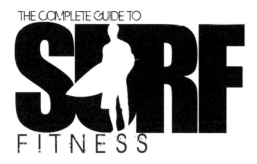

THE COMPLETE GUIDE TO SURF FITNESS

BY LEE STANBURY

ISBN 978-0-9523646-6-5

Published by Orca Publications Limited,
Berry Road Studios, Berry Road, Newquay, TR7 1AT,
United Kingdom.   +44 (0) 1637 878074 www.orcasurf.co.uk

Printed in China.

THIS BOOK WOULDN'T HAVE BEEN POSSIBLE WITHOUT THE HELP AND SUPPORT OF THE FOLLOWING PEOPLE

DESIGN AND PHOTOGRAPHY
BEN HARRIS   www.visualammo.co.uk

SURF PHOTOGRAPHY
TONY PLANT, GEOFF TYDEMAN , MIKE SEARLE, ROGER SHARP

EDITORIAL CONSULTANT
MIKE SEARLE

MODEL/SURFER
ALEX GOLLAY - AKA FELIX

FEATURED SURFERS
BEN SKINNER - SOPHIE SKINNER - LEE BARTLETT - OLI ADAMS - TASSY SWALLOW

THANKS TO:
W.E. SURFBOARDS   EDD STANBURY ARTIST   MALCOLM BALL SNUGG WETSUITS

JON BAXENDALE WWW.A1SURF.CO.UK   HAGER-VOR SURF WWW.HAGERVOR.CO.UK

CARVE SURF MAGAZINE WWW.ORCASURF.CO.UK

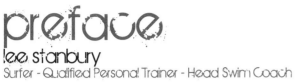

preface
lee stanbury
Surfer - Qualified Personal Trainer - Head Swim Coach

As a former competitive swimmer and world biathlete with 20 years experience in the health and fitness industry, I understand how my fitness and the type of training I do can affect my surfing. Over the last few years I've developed a series of exercises that specifically target areas that aid my surfing performance. As a direct result my surfing movements have become more dynamic and my endurance and paddle power are better than they've ever been.

Land-based training for surfers has now become a passion of mine. I'm always looking for that little edge that's going to aid my surfing and help any other surfers along the way too.

There's no question that regular land-based training will improve your surfing. This book has been put together to fully open up the endless types of training available to any surfer from beginner to pro. As the strength and conditioning coach for top British surfers Ben Skinner (2009 European longboard champion) and Oli Adams, I have an ideal insight into what helps an athlete at the top of their game achieve that next level of fitness.

I will outline the basic principles of how to gain more strength, endurance and power in your surfing and give you a straightforward basic understanding to help you stay injury free and ready for whatever the ocean can throw at you.

www.cornwallpersonaltraining.co.uk

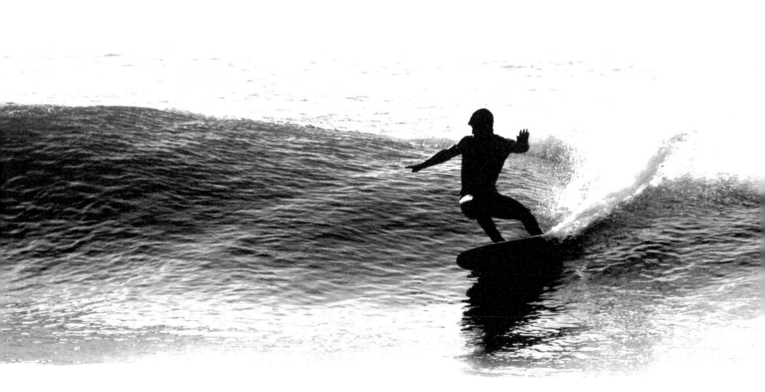

CONTENTS

BEFORE YOU START

Before taking up any new exercise programme we strongly advise
that you seek medical advice if you suffer from any medical condition
or have any injuries that may put you at risk from further injury.

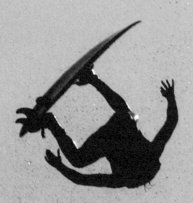

IMAGE BY TONY PLANT

INTRODUCTION

IN THIS BOOK YOU WILL FIND EXERCISES THAT WILL ENHANCE YOUR SURFING

For many of you, driving down the road, suiting up and paddling out regularly is not an option. This book can help you maintain your surfing fitness so when you are able to surf you are stronger, fitter and have more explosive power.

The exercises in this book will give you some idea of the vast range of training types available to the surfer.

Surfing is a sport, and like any sport there is a vast range of exercises that can improve your performance. This book will help give you a basic understanding of how to plan a constructive weekly training session that can be done practically anywhere, from your home to the gym.

Today, as we learn how to push the limits further and further, new exercises are being developed to reach the fitness levels required. In this first book we will touch on just a few of them, but the effect on your fitness will amaze you.

All the exercises in this book have been put together with the following in mind...

SURF LONGER, CATCH MORE WAVES AND BOOST YOUR PERFORMANCE DOWN THE LINE!

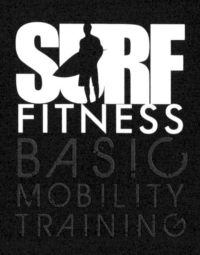

SURF
FITNESS
BASIC
MOBILITY
TRAINING

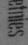

IMPORTANT

Remember, when
undertaking any of the
exercises in this section,
stay within your normal
range of motion.

Care must be taken with all
exercise. By going too fast
initially you risk injuring
yourself before you've
even got in the water!

lee bartlett

BASIC MOBILITY
TRAINING

PRE-SURF MOBILITY EXERCISES

Many surfers prepare for a surf by carrying out routine stretching exercises. It is important to remember that stretching helps to improve your static (non-moving) flexibility and may not do such a good job at preparing your body to move quickly and efficiently. This is why some dynamic mobility work before each surf can help.

Most sports involve some form of strenuous activity and surfing is no different. By using mobility exercises as well as drills that stimulate your nervous system, muscles, tendons and joints in a dynamic manner, your performance can be improved.

POST-SURF STATIC STRETCHES

Static stretches that do not involve much movement are simply elongating a particular muscle or muscle group. They do have a place in your training programme and surfing, but their value and proper usage are often misunderstood. It's often better to use stretches after you've finished exercising or a surf.

A ten minute stretch after a surf can leave you feeling refreshed the following day and ready for another session, instead of feeling like a cardboard cut out with your shoulders and back screaming "no more!"

IMPORTANT TO REMEMBER

When undertaking any pre-exercise mobility movements, it is important to use a smooth controlled motion. You should start with small movements and only use a larger range of movement as your reps progress.

AS YOU WARM UP YOU SHOULD GRADUALLY INCREASE YOUR SPEED TO MAKE YOUR MOVEMENTS MORE DYNAMIC

1 NECK MOBILITY — 3 MOVEMENTS

FORWARDS — FLEXION

THE START POSITION
Slowly tilt your head forward, tucking your chin into your chest. If this causes you any discomfort refrain from stretching any further. Lift your chin upwards, leaning your head back as far as possible.

Repeat this 5-6 times.

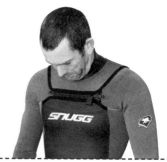

SIDEWAYS — LATERAL FLEXION

THE START POSITION
Tilt your head to the left, lowering your left ear towards your left shoulder in a slow and controlled motion. Then tilt your head to the right, lowering your right ear towards your right shoulder.

Hold each for 10 seconds and repeat.

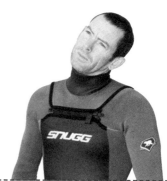

ROTATION

THE START POSITION
Turn your chin laterally towards your left shoulder, then rotate towards your right shoulder and continue rotating fully through 360°.

Repeat this 5-6 times.

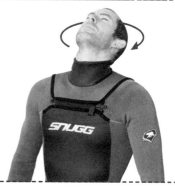

2 TWISTS

THE START POSITION

Stand with your feet hip width apart and your arms extended straight out in front of you. Keeping your feet facing forwards, twist your torso and hips to the right, shifting your weight on to your right foot. Then twist your torso to the left while shifting your weight to your left foot.

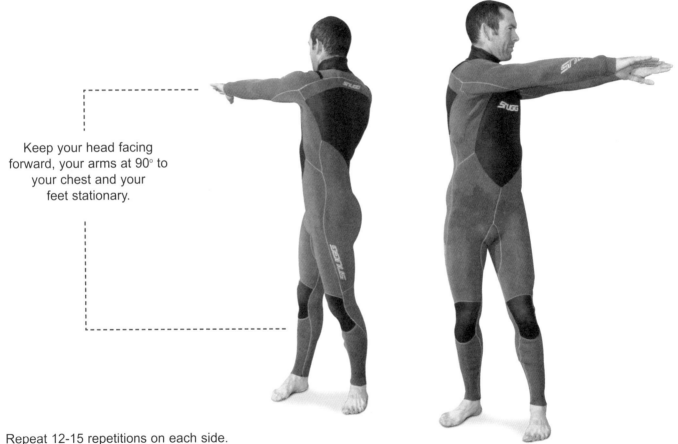

Keep your head facing forward, your arms at 90° to your chest and your feet stationary.

Repeat 12-15 repetitions on each side.

TRY NOT TO TURN YOUR HEAD WHILE TWISTING AND ALWAYS KEEP YOUR MOVEMENTS SLOW AND CONTROLLED

3 LEG SWINGS

THE START POSITION
Stand with your feet hip width apart and place your hands on your hips to help you balance. Keeping your back straight and your head up, swing your right leg forward to its fullest comfortable extent and let it swing backwards extending it behind you, completing a full range of movement.

Keeping your head up and looking straight ahead will help you to keep your balance

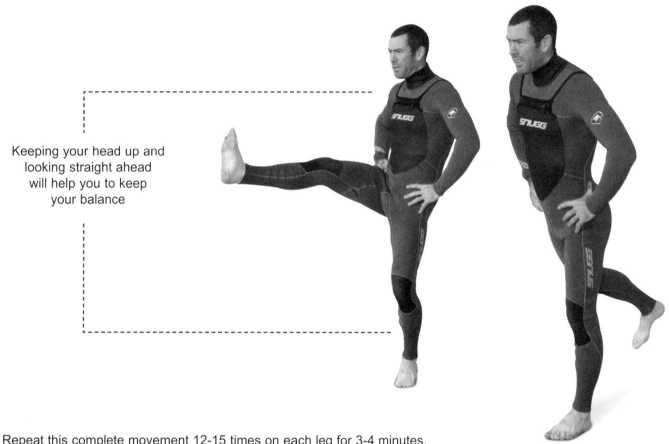

Repeat this complete movement 12-15 times on each leg for 3-4 minutes.

IT IS IMPORTANT NOT TO OVER EXTEND YOUR LEGS AND ALWAYS KEEP YOUR MOVEMENTS SLOW AND CONTROLLED

BASIC MOBILITY EXERCISES

4 ANKLE ROTATIONS

THE START POSITION
Stand with your feet hip width apart and your hands on your hips. Extend your left leg out in front of you, point your toes and rotate your foot at the ankle, drawing a circle in the air with your toes.

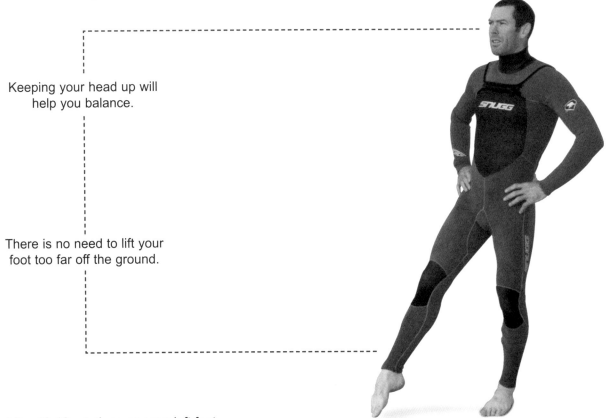

Keeping your head up will help you balance.

There is no need to lift your foot too far off the ground.

After 10-12 rotations on your left foot, change over to the right leg and repeat.

REMEMBER TO ALWAYS KEEP YOUR MOVEMENTS SLOW AND CONTROLLED

5 CHICKEN WINGS TO A PADDLE

THE START POSITION
Start by standing with your feet hip width apart. Tuck your hands into your shoulders to make 'chicken wings'. Slowly rotate your arms at your shoulders 12-15 times forwards and then 12-15 times backwards.

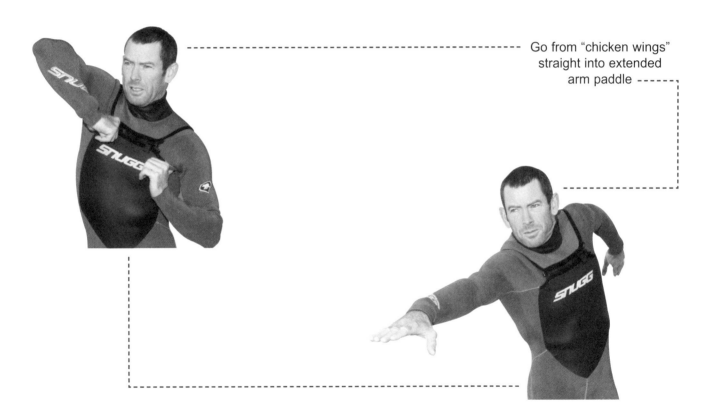

Go from "chicken wings" straight into extended arm paddle

Move straight from chicken wings into an extended arm paddle (front crawl) movement for a further 12-15 times.

KEEP YOUR MOVEMENTS SLOW AND CONTROLLED

6 BASIC ARM SWINGS

THE START POSITION
Swing your right arm forwards, rotating at the shoulder in one slow controlled movement and completing a full 360° rotation.

Basic arm swings can also be done backwards, again rotating your arm at the shoulder in one slow controlled movement through a full 360°.

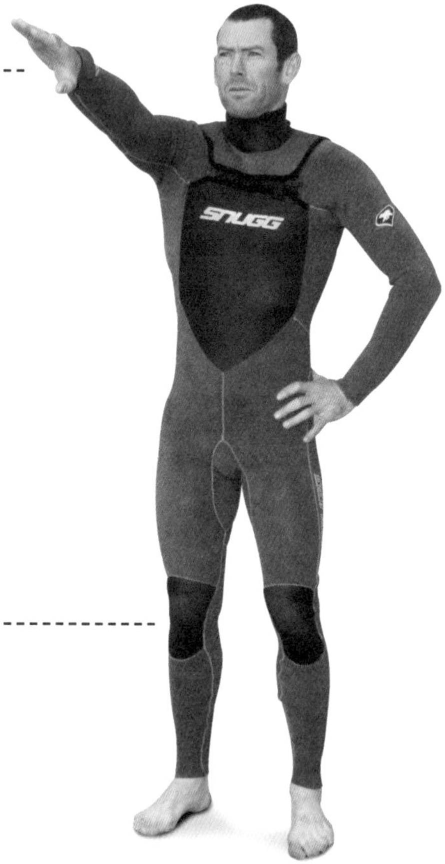

Keep your body facing
forwards and don't
overstretch your shoulder
during the rotation

Complete 15-20 forward rotations on each arm
and then the same backwards.

REMEMBER TO ALWAYS KEEP YOUR MOVEMENTS SLOW AND CONTROLLED

7 DOUBLE ARM SWINGS

THE START POSITION
Stand with your feet hip width apart facing forwards. Simultaneously swing both of your arms forwards, rotating them at the shoulder in one slow controlled movement through a full 360°.

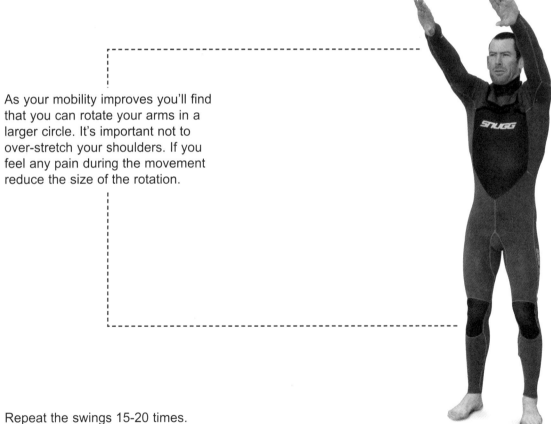

As your mobility improves you'll find that you can rotate your arms in a larger circle. It's important not to over-stretch your shoulders. If you feel any pain during the movement reduce the size of the rotation.

Repeat the swings 15-20 times.

THIS EXERCISE SHOULD NOT BE DONE IN REVERSE.

MUSCLES OF THE BODY A few of the muscles that make up the body

1 DELTOID

2 PECTORALIS MAJOR

3 BICEPS

4 SERRATUS ANTERIOR

5 BRACHIALIS

6 ABDOMINAL OBLIQUE

7 RECTUS ABDOMINIS

8 ADDUCTOR BREVIS

9 VASTUS LATERALIS

10 RECTUS FEMORIS

11 SOLEUS

12 TIBIALIS ANTERIOR

13 EXTENSOR DIGITORUM

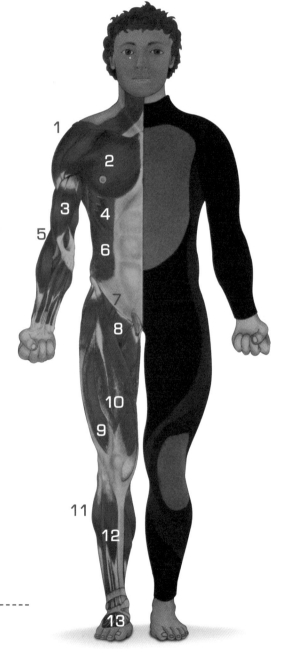

MUSCLE FUNCTIONS

DELTOIDS - Aid paddling, used in lifting movements

PECTORALIS MAJOR - Aids your pop up and paddle power

ABDOMINAL OBLIQUES - Aid any diagonal torso movements

RECTUS ABDOMINIS - Aids stability, posture and allows forward movement

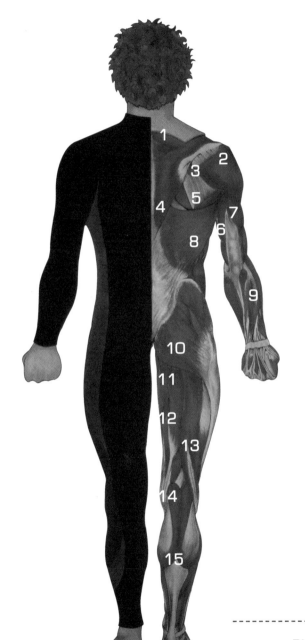

1 TRAPEZIUS

2 DELTOID

3 INFRASPINATUS

4 RHOMBOID

5 SUPRASPINATUS

6 TRICEPS - LONGHEAD

7 TRICEPS - LATERAL HEAD

8 LATISSIMUS DORSI

9 FLEXOR DIGTORUM

10 GLUTEUS MAXIMUS

11 ADDUCTOR MAGNUS

12 GRACILIS

13 BICEPS FEMORIS

14 SARTORIUS

15 GASTROCNEMIUS

MUSCLE FUNCTIONS

RHOMBOID - Aids paddle movements, also helps protect the spine

LATISSIMUS DORSI - Aids paddle power and body lowering movements

GLUTEUS MAXIMUS - Aids stability whilst turning your board

TRICEPS - Aid paddle power, allow you to straighten your arms against pressure

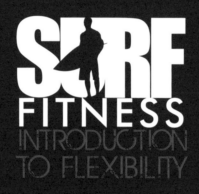

SURF
FITNESS
INTRODUCTION
TO FLEXIBILITY

FLEXIBILITY IS KEY TO ANY SURFER

Increasing your flexibility will help you
take your surfing to the next level"

lee bartlett

FLEXIBILITY

INTRODUCTION

INTRODUCTION TO FLEXIBILITY

WARM UP STRETCHING AND MOBILITY

WHAT IS FLEXIBILITY?

Flexibility is the ability to perform a joint action through a range of movement. Improving mobility and flexibility for surfing has become an essential part of any surfer's regime.This acceptance has come through greater understanding and awareness of the fact that increasing your joint flexibility increases your joints' potential to produce a more effective range of movement (ROM) while surfing or exercising, which can enhance your overall performance.

In addition to the above, increasing a joint's flexibility reduces the potential risk of injury to that joint. By increasing the flexibility of your joints you put less strain on the muscles surrounding them than you would if the joint was stiff.

WHY IS FLEXIBILITY IMPORTANT?

In the body's movements there are two groups of muscles at work: the antagonist muscles (muscles which relax and lengthen to allow a movement to occur) and the agonist muscles (muscles whose contraction is directly responsible for the movement of a part of the body). As a surfer the objective of flexibility training is to improve the range of movement within these muscle groups.

If you are stretching correctly you should feel mild discomfort in the antagonistic muscles. Remember, if you feel pain or a sharp stabbing sensation then it is advisable that you stop!

The human body responds best when it is warm. You should consider this when undertaking flexibility exercises. Warming the body correctly will allow muscles and joints to be taken through their correct range of movement.

TYPES OF STRETCHING

There are many different types of stretching available to the surfer

STATIC STRETCHING

This is one of the most well-known forms of basic stretching, which involves gradually easing into the stretch position and holding it. The amount of time you spend on a static stretch really depends on your objectives. If you are spending time on stretching as a cool down then 10-15 seconds should be enough, but if you are stretching to improve your ROM and your mobility then you should hold the stretches for 30 seconds or more.

BALLISTIC STRETCHING

Ballistic stretching can be beneficial just before a surf session, but take care! This form of stretching uses the momentum of the body or a limb in an attempt to force it beyond its normal range of movement. Dynamic stretching, for example arm swings (see basic mobility exercises), will slowly ease your body into a state where you can take advantage of its full range of movements. As mentioned before, dynamic and ballistic movements should always be done with care and starting off at half speed is advisable.

PASSIVE STRETCHING

This is also know as relaxed stretching or as static-passive stretching. In this form of stretching you assume a stretch position and hold it with some other part of your body, or with the assistance of a training partner or coach.

ASSISTED/DEVELOPMENTAL STRETCHING

Following on from passive stretching, assisted stretching involves the assistance of a partner who is experienced and understands the principles of assisted stretching. With partner stretching, your partner assists you in maintaining the stretch position, or they can help ease you into the stretch position. When involved in partner stretching you should be fully relaxed throughout the exercise. This type of flexibility training can be used for developing your flexibility to much higher levels and is otherwise known as developmental flexibility.

WHEN SHOULD I DO MOST OF MY STRETCHING OR FLEXIBILITY WORK?

Over the last few years there has been much research into flexibility and the best time to stretch.

It is widely believed that lengthy static stretching before activity may cause a temporary decrease in strength and power. It is important for athletes who participate in sports that require power and explosiveness, like surfers, to be fully aware of this fact as it may affect your mobility and performance.

If you are just about to hit the water for a wave or about to run or swim it may be of more benefit to warm up with some light aerobic and mobility activity and then do static stretches. Any stretching pre-surf should be very light and short.

BY DOING A CONSTRUCTIVE STRETCHING AND FLEXIBILITY SESSION AFTER YOUR SURF OR WORKOUT YOU WILL NOT COMPROMISE YOUR STRENGTH AND POWER.

1 HIP - FLEXORS
Specifically stretches the top of your thighs

THE START POSITION
Step forwards on your right leg and gently lower your left leg until you feel a mild stretch at the top of your left thigh; hold this position. Rest both hands on your right leg and keep your back as straight as possible.

Keep your head up and
your back straight
throughout the stretch

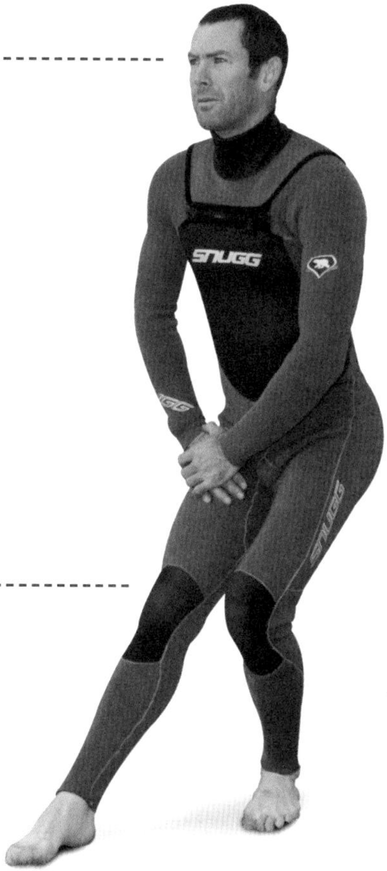

Repeat this for 12-15 reps then switch and repeat on the opposite leg.

AIDS INJURY PREVENTION

2 HAMSTRINGS

Stretches the back of your legs.

THE START POSITION

Extend your right leg out in front of you with your heel on the floor and your toes pointing upwards. Bend your left leg slightly, lowering your body towards the floor. You can support yourself by placing your hands on your bent leg. Slowly lean forwards until you feel a mild stretch in the hamstring of your extended leg.

It's really easy to over-stretch during stretching sessions. If you feel any pain at any point during the stretch ease off until you feel comfortable.

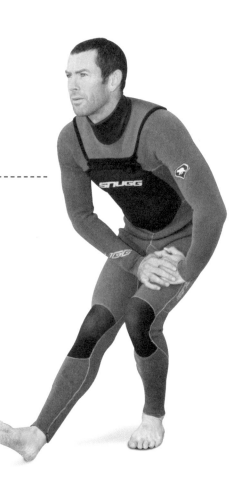

Keep your head up and your back straight throughout the stretch.

Repeat this for 12-15 reps then switch and repeat on the opposite leg.

AIDS INJURY PREVENTION

3 ERECTOR SPINE

This will stretch the muscles around the spine.

THE START POSITION

Place your feet hip width apart and slowly bend your knees. Lean forwards placing your hands just above your knees to support your back. Gently round your spine and hold this stretch position.

Don't over-stretch your back. If you feel any pain ease off slightly.

KEEP YOUR MOVEMENTS SLOW AND CONTROLLED THROUGHOUT THE STRETCH

Repeat this for 12-15 reps holding each stretch for approximately 20 seconds.

AIDS INJURY PREVENTION

4 QUADRICEPS

Stretches the front of your legs.

THE START POSITION

Slightly bend your supporting leg and draw the heel of the opposite foot towards your bottom. Remember to maintain an upright body position during the stretch and make sure your hips are facing forwards.

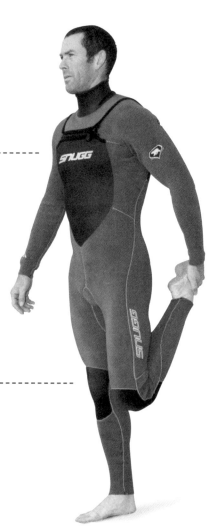

You can use a wall or some other form of support for this stretch.

Repeat this for 12-15 reps then switch and repeat on the opposite leg.

AIDS INJURY PREVENTION

5 LATISSIMUS DORSI/OBLIQUES
This will specifically stretch your mid-back and sides.

THE START POSITION
Place your feet slightly wider than hip width apart and slightly bend your knees. Arch your right arm over your head, keeping it slightly bent with your palm facing out. Making sure you keep your hips facing forwards.

As with all stretches, don't bounce! Keep your movements slow and controlled.

Repeat this for 12-15 reps then switch and repeat on the opposite side.

AIDS INJURY PREVENTION

6 ADDUCTORS

This will stretch the inside of your legs.

THE START POSITION

Stand with your feet slightly wider than hip width apart. Bend your right knee as far as you feel comfortable, placing your hands on your thighs to help you balance. You should feel the stretch through the inner thigh of your left leg.

Keep your back straight, your head level and your shoulders facing forwards.

Repeat this for 12-15 reps then switch and repeat on the opposite side.

AIDS INJURY PREVENTION

Images of surfing in the UK

Ben Skinner surfing in Cornwall

Photography by Geoff Tydeman

EDITORIAL   ADVERTISING   PORTFOLIOS

email: *geoff.tydeman@hotmail.co.uk*
web: *http://gtimages.ifp3.com*

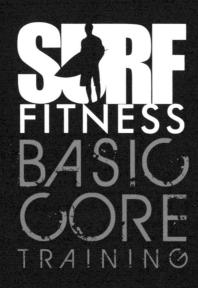

SURF FITNESS
BASIC CORE TRAINING

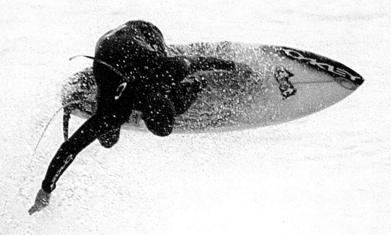

"CORE TRAINING ON A REGULAR BASIS HAS ADDED NEW STRENGTH TO MY SURFING"

Ali Adams
Oakley team rider

BASIC CORE
TRAINING

CORE STABILITY TRAINING

Core stability training is a great start if you are looking at undertaking a new exercise programme. It can be completely cost free and can be done anywhere at any time. Additional core strength can be gained by implementing the use of a variety of different pieces of equipment.

This type of training is highly beneficial to any surfer, aiding performance and injury prevention. Core muscles are the foundation for all of the body's movements. The muscles of the abdominal area and torso help stabilise the spine and provide a solid foundation for many surfing movements.

Many surfers are now familiar with the term core stability and there

are many forms of core training available today for surfers to tap into. The aim of core strength training is to increase the efficiency of the smaller, deeper, stabilising muscles which help you balance, such as the transverse abdominals which lie deep within your abdominal area.

Core strength exercises range in difficulty from the beginner through to the advanced, which do require some previous experience with exercise balls and exercise equipment.

If you are new to stability and core training it is advised that you avoid any exercise that causes pain or you are unsure of. It's always best to see your doctor if you have any injuries or conditions.

TOP TIP

BODY POSITION
Your spine should be in a neutral position. A neutral position for your spine is one in which your lower back is naturally curved, not flattened or arched. This will put your pelvis in a stress-free position and also activates your abdominals, particularly your transverse abdominals.

1 THE SIDE PLANK

The plank is a static exercise that will strengthen the core, back and shoulders. It's a good stabilising exercise that specifically targets the trunk, which is important to surfing fitness. The advantage of this exercise is that it can be done anywhere without equipment.

THE START POSITION

Begin by lifting your body off the ground, balancing on one forearm and the side of your foot. Your arm should be at 90^0 to your body and your shoulder should be over your elbow.

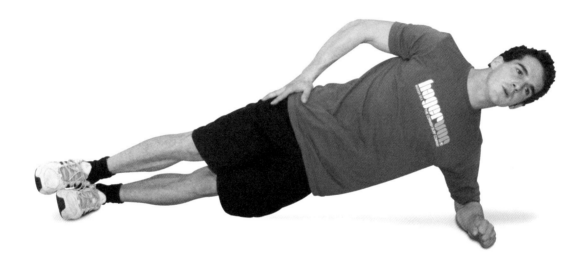

Making sure you are well balanced and comfortable, contract your abdominals and relax your shoulders. Try to keep a good body alignment and your neck straight. If you are exercising on a hard floor try to use a mat to avoid damage to your forearms and feet.

No movement — the longer you hold, the stronger you get!

IMPROVES STABILITY DURING PADDLING, STRENGTHENS THE OBLIQUES, ABDOMINALS, BACK AND SHOULDERS

2 THE FRONT PLANK

Exercise for stability during paddling.

The front plank is a static exercise that will strengthen your abdominals, back and shoulders. It specifically strengthens the transverse abdominals which are the deepest layer of abdominal muscle that wraps around your whole mid-section.

As previously suggested, before you start pay attention to the surface your exercising on. You should try to exercise on a cushioned non-slip surface where possible to avoid injury.

THE START POSITION

Lift your body completely off the ground, transferring your bodyweight onto your elbows and toes. Contract your abdominals and relax your shoulders.

Try to maintain a good straight body alignment throughout. Keep breathing easily and relax your neck.

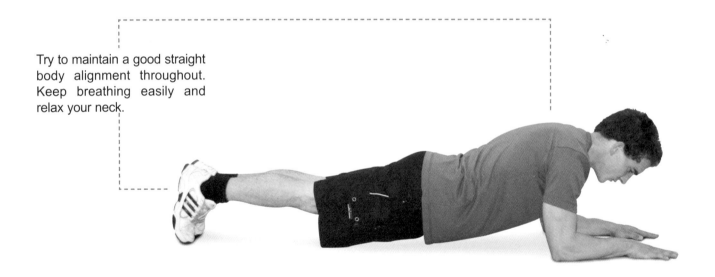

Hold the exercise for as long as you can and contract your abdominals constantly throughout the exercise.

IMPROVES STABILITY DURING PADDLING, STRENGTHENS ABDOMINALS, BACK AND SHOULDERS AND ADDS A REAL BOOST TO YOUR CORE STRENGTH.

3 SCISSOR PLANK

Advanced exercise for stability during paddling.

THE START POSITION

Start the scissor plank in the front plank position. With your elbows in line with your shoulders and keeping your abdominals tight, lift one leg.

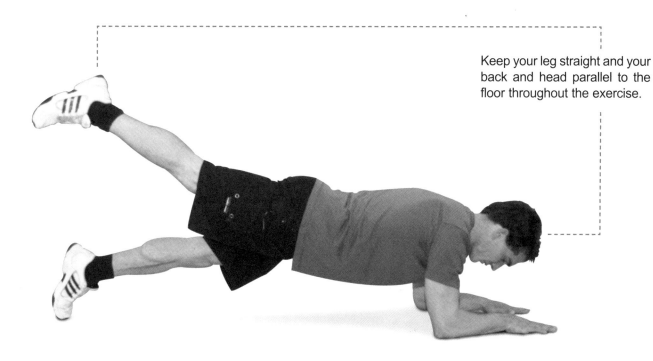

Keep your leg straight and your back and head parallel to the floor throughout the exercise.

Repeat this as many times as you can. Be sure to contract your abdominals constantly throughout the exercise.

IMPROVES YOUR TRANSVERSE ABDOMINALS, YOUR BALANCE & CO-ORDINATION

BASIC ABDOMINAL EXERCISES

1 SLOW AND CONTROLLED CRUNCHES
Exercise for strength during paddling.

This is a very basic crunch, so if you are not that strong in the abdominal area this is a good starting exercise to build on.

THE START POSITION
Lie on your back with your knees bent and your feet flat on the floor. Place your hands by your ears and curl your shoulders forwards keeping your lower back on the floor. Breathe out as you lift and breathe in as you lower back down to the start position.

Try to maintain a good body alignment throughout. Keep breathing easy, relax your neck and keep your feet flat on the floor.

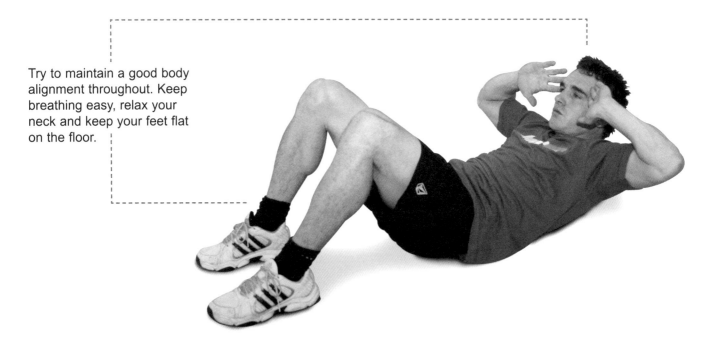

Keep a space the size of a tennis ball under your chin. Each rep should take about 2-3 seconds, repeat 3 sets of 10 reps initially and increase with time.

MUSCLES WORKED —RECTUS ABDOMINIS

2 BASIC CRUNCH WITH LEGS IN THE AIR

Exercise for strength during paddling and all surfing movements.

This exercise targets the lower part of the abdominals. By targeting a specific muscle group it puts less strain on the neck, reducing the risk of injury.

THE START POSITION

Lie on your back with your hands by your ears and your legs straight up in the air. Cross your legs to stabilise the movement. Tighten your lower abdominals and with short bursts of effort simultaneously crunch up towards your knees.

You should try to keep your legs in the same position throughout. During the entire exercise, maintain a slow and controlled movement and try not to let your shoulder blades touch the floor.

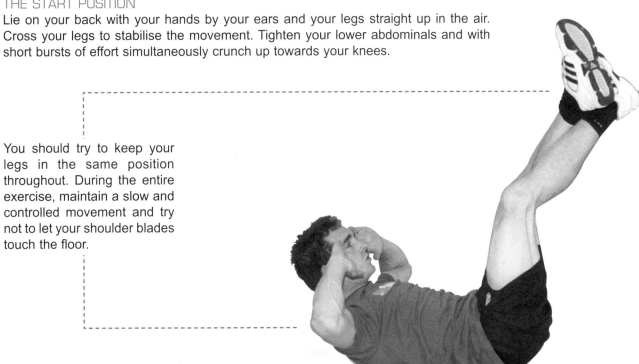

Each rep should take about 2-3 seconds. Repeat 3 sets of 10 reps initially and increase with time.

MUSCLES WORKED — RECTUS ABDOMINIS

ABDOMINAL EXERCISES

1 LEGS UP ON THE BALL CRUNCHES
Aids paddling strength.

THE START POSITION
Lie on your back with your legs flexed and your feet on the ball. Roll your shoulders forward lifting them off the floor. Extend your arms and position your hands on the outside of each knee.

Hold at the top of the crunch for around 2-3 seconds before relaxing back down to the floor.

Try to maintain a good body alignment throughout. Keep your breathing easy and your neck relaxed.

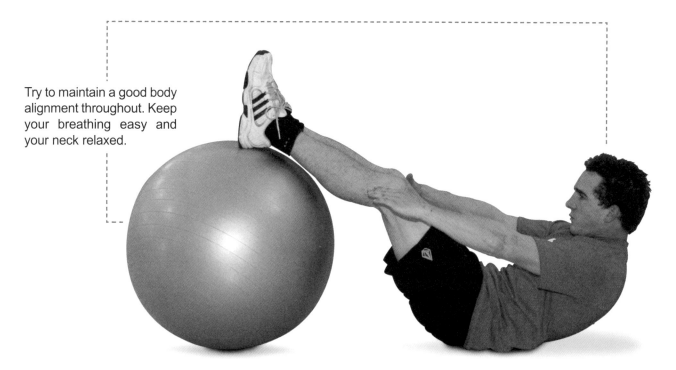

Breathe in as you roll your shoulders forwards and breathe out as you relax back down. Maintain slow controlled movements throughout the exercise.

MUSCLES WORKED —RECTUS ABDOMINIS

2 SWISS BALL CRUNCH

THE START POSITION

Lie on the ball with your knees bent at 90° Extend your arms with hands on top of your thighs. Hold for 2-3 seconds. Position yourself so that your mid back and upper pelvis are resting against the ball. Your feet should be shoulder width apart.

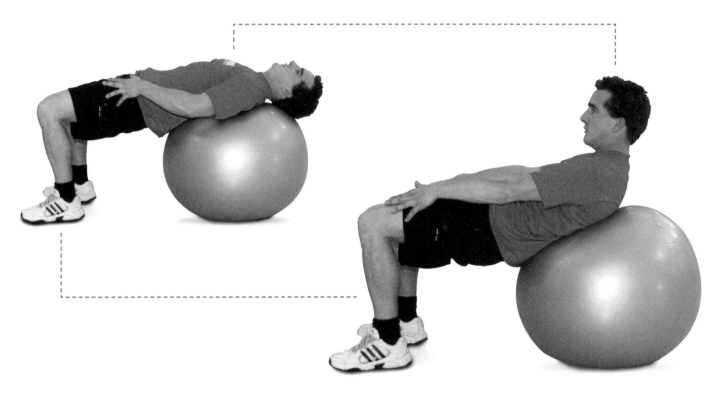

Tighten your abdominal muscles to flex your midsection, then lift your shoulders forwards as you reach your hands towards your knees. Hold for 2-3 seconds.

STABILISES YOUR UPPER BODY DURING PADDLING AND JUST BEFORE THE POP-UP

ABDOMINAL EXERCISES

MUSCLE MAKE-UP OF YOUR CORE STRENGTH

1. TRANSVERSE ABDOMINALS

This is the flat sheath of muscle that lies under the main rectus abdominis and runs across the torso. They also give support to the internal organs and play a major role in most surfing movements from paddling to just sitting on your board waiting for that next set!

2 .EXTERNAL OBLIQUES

These cover the front and side of your abdomen and run diagonally from the lowest part of the ribs to the pelvis forming a V shape. These muscles help bend the torso sideways and rotate it to the opposite side when flexing forwards.

3. INTERNAL OBLIQUES

These lie directly underneath the external obliques but run in the opposite direction. They assist in bending the rectus abdominis forwards. The external and internal obliques play a major role in many surfing movements, from basic bottom turns to a full super-fast roundhouse movement!

4. RECTUS ABDOMINIS

More commonly known as the six pack! We all have them but most are covered with a percentage of fat, only totally visible to the lucky few with low body fat. These long slender muscles run vertically down your abdomen from the lowest part of your ribs to your pelvic bone. This muscle assists in flexing the torso forwards.

TOP TIP

BODY POSITION
If you are looking to increase your abdominal strength and gain additional core stability, training 2 or 3 times a week is essential. Abdominals, like any muscle, can benefit from a constructive cool down stretch after any exercise or abdominal workout.

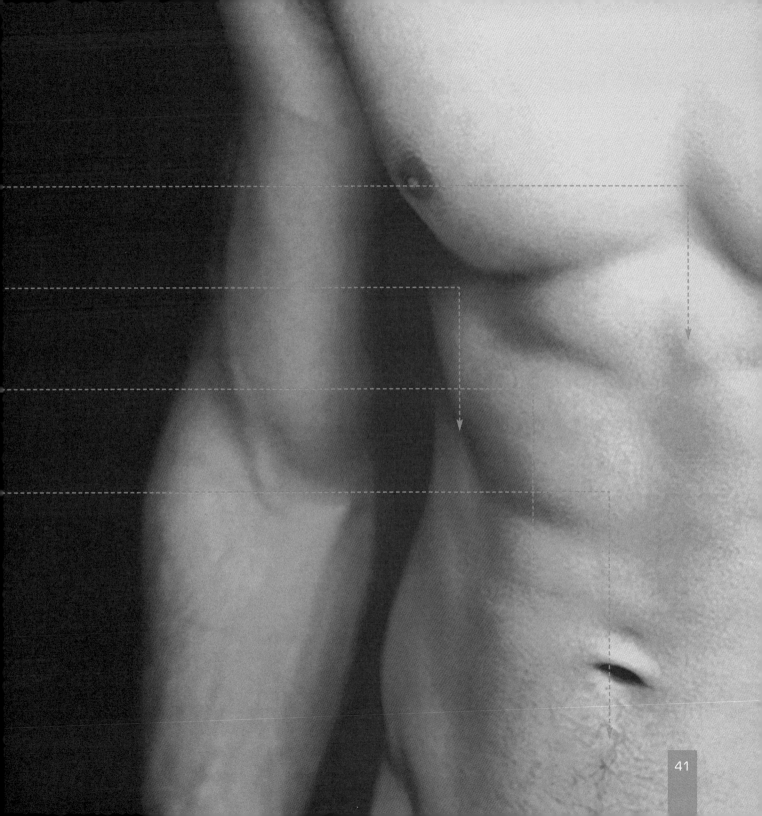

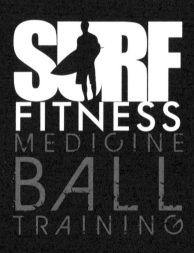

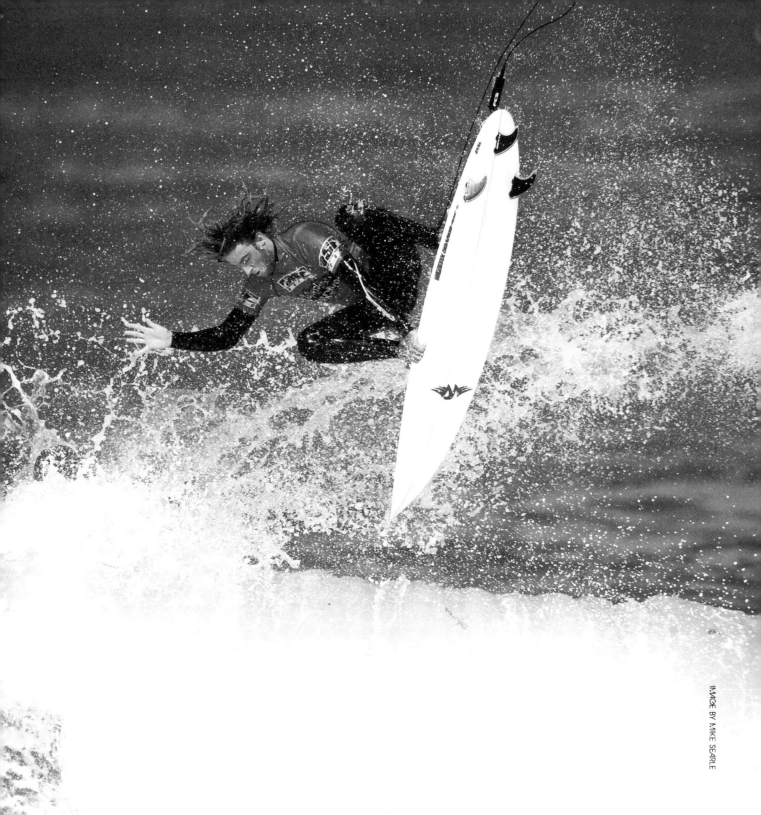

MEDICINE BALL

TRAINING

MEDICINE BALL FOR SURFING STRENGTH

For surfers seriously training hard to maintain high levels of fitness, the medicine ball or Xerball can be a fantastic training tool. The medicine ball has been around for some time. Used in the past by elite athletes and coaches, in today's growing fitness industry it is commonly used and can play a key role in any surfer's training programme.

By using a medicine ball in your training programme you will improve the strength in your tendons, ligaments and bones, improve your core strength and benefit from a great form of resistance training.

BASIC MEDICINE BALL GUIDELINES

Always warm up before using the medicine ball. An 8-10 minute warm up will help all medicine ball movements to be fluent and free flowing.

You should perform a minimum of 10-12 sperate exercises that will train all the major muscle groups.

Every exercise should be performed through a full range of motion in a controlled manner.

One of your main goals as a surfer is to increase muscular endurance. Performing straight repetitions for 60 seconds will mean a higher level of fitness.

Initially use a lighter weight ball and gradually progress to a ball that's a bit heavier.

Working at a fast tempo is important but take care that speed does not affect your technique.

Seek a professional's advice about medicine ball training as there are many types of programmes available that target different areas.

ADDITIONAL BENEFITS TO MEDICINE BALL TRAINING

Medicine ball training is a great way to get into shape for surfing. It increases muscle mass, bone mass and connective tissue thickness, as well as associated increases in muscle strength and endurance.

With regular training using medicine balls, additional strength gains can also positively affect your posture and body mechanics. This will help decrease the risk of overuse injuries.

Medicine balls come in a variety of weights and materials. It's important that you use a ball you are comfortable with to exercise.

TOP TIP
REASONS TO USE A MEDICINE BALL FOR TRAINING

- Increased contractile muscle strength and increased muscle endurance.

- Increased metabolism.

- Increased calorie burning.

- Improved posture.

- Aids injury prevention for your muscles and joints.

MEDICINE BALL EXERCISES

1 MEDICINE BALL PRESS-UP SHUFFLES

As a beginner you should build up your strength with basic press-ups before progressing to more advanced exercises.

THE START POSITION
Get into a press-up position with your left hand on the medicine ball and your right hand on the ground. Maintain a straight back and bend your elbows to lower yourself until your chest is on the medicine ball. Push up with both hands to the start position.

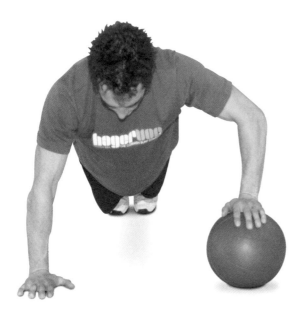
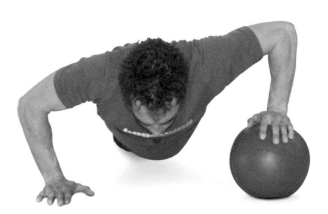

ADVANCING THE EXERCISE
Explosively push back up off the medicine ball with enough force to lift your hands off the ball and the floor. As you lift off the ball, pass it to your other hand landing with your opposite hand on the ball.

Do 5 sets of 5 reps on each side.

GREAT FOR BUILDING UPPER BODY STRENGTH

2 MEDICINE BALL THROWS

THE START POSITION

Sit upright facing your training partner with your legs bent and your feet flat on the floor in front of you. Hold the medicine ball above your head and slowly lean backwards keeping your legs and feet in the same position. Try to keep your shoulders and head from touching the floor.

As you sit back up, throw the ball as far as you can forwards to your partner. Keep your arms fully extended, your abdominals tight and your movements slow and controlled.

MAKE SURE YOU USE A WEIGHT YOU ARE BOTH COMFORTABLE WITH

Do 4-5 sets of 10-12 throws with a short rest between each set.

GREAT FOR CORE AND ABDOMINAL STRENGTH

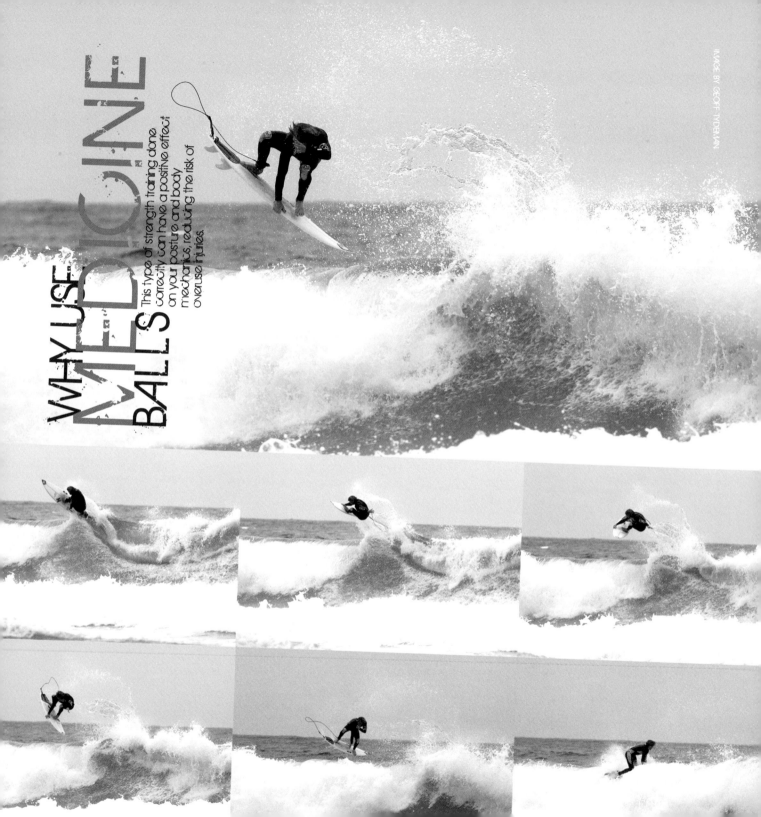

WHY USE MEDICINE BALLS

This type of strength training done correctly can have a positive effect on your posture and body mechanics, reducing the risk of overuse injuries.

3 STANDING TORSO TWIST

THE START POSITION
Stand back to back about 1 metre apart with your hips facing forward. Pass the ball to one another by twisting your torso. Make sure you keep your hips facing forwards and your feet in the same position.

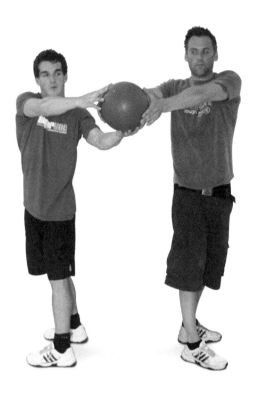 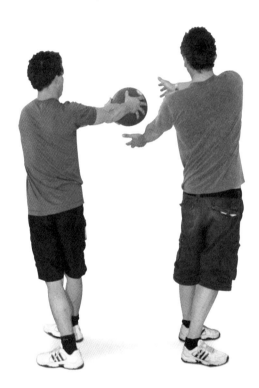

This exercise can also be done sitting on the floor back to back with your legs extended out in front of you.

ADVANCING THE EXERCISE
Try repeating the movement on your own, sat on the floor with your legs extended and raised about 6 inches.

GREAT FOR STRENGTHENING MID SECTION

MEDICINE BALL - TRAINING THE LEGS

1 ALTERNATING LUNGE WITH MEDICINE BALL

THE START POSITION
Stand with your feet about hip width apart. Take a step forwards with your left foot and bend your knee until your left thigh is parallel to the floor.

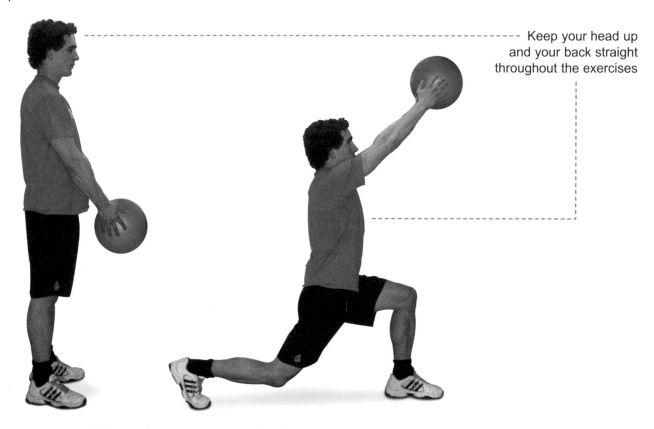

Keep your head up and your back straight throughout the exercises

During this movement it is very important that your back remains straight and you avoid touching the floor with your knee. As the leading leg steps forward lift the medicine ball above your head with extended arms.

TRY DOING THE SAME MOVEMENT WHILST WALKING FORWARDS IN A STRAIGHT LINE UNTIL YOU REACH FAILURE

2 THE MEDICINE BALL SQUAT

THE START POSITION

Standing with your feet slightly wider than hip width apart, bend your hips and knees to lower yourself into a sitting position. As you do this raise the medicine ball up to shoulder level then repeat to failure. Maintain a straight back throughout the movement.

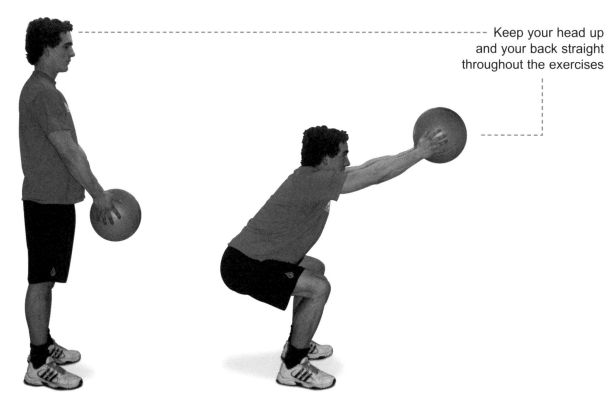

Keep your head up and your back straight throughout the exercises

To start, try the movements without the medicine ball. Once your balance has improved introduce the ball. The medicine ball adds extra resistance and the shoulders get a workout too!

GREAT FOR STRENGTHENING YOUR THIGHS

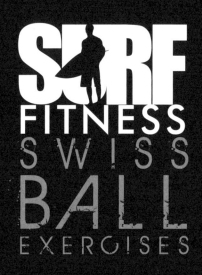

**SURF
FITNESS
SWISS
BALL
EXERCISES**

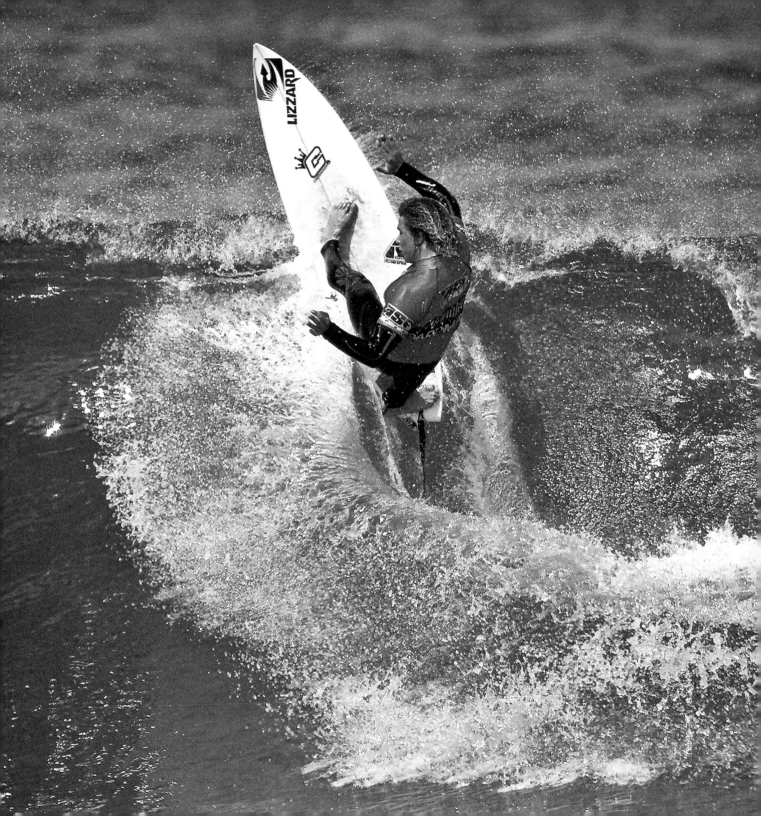

SWISS BALL
EXERCISES

THE SWISS BALL
FOR SURFING STRENGTH

THE BENEFITS

The benefits of the Swiss ball in developing body strength are vast, not only in surfing but in all sports. There are a whole range of exercises available to the surfer to suit all abilities, from beginners to the more advanced. Technique while training with the Swiss ball is vital so before any Swiss ball training seek the advice of a trained professional.

By using the Swiss ball for surf fitness and strength you will gain many physical benefits such as improved back strength, improved posture, core strength and stability, good muscle balance and improved mobility.

Working with the Swiss ball on a weekly basis will strengthen the structures of the back directly responsible for spinal health and injury prevention. Whilst using the ball you will build good posture awareness and strength. This means that your abdominal and spinal muscles are worked and therefore strengthened. This is a major factor within total surfing fitness.

Simply by exercising with light weights whilst using the ball you are recruiting several more muscle groups, some of which you may never have felt before. By strengthening all of these muscle groups you will gain extra surfing strength.

BASIC GUIDELINES FOR SWISS BALL USE

Buy or use a Swiss ball that is the right size for your height. There are numerous exercise balls on the market and they vary in colour, size and quality. Cheaper balls are often slippery, making them less safe in certain positions.

TOP TIP

THINGS TO REMEMBER

- Start off slowly and, as your strength increases, increase your speed.

- Maintain control and good posture throughout the exercise.

- Work hard on precision and not so much on speed.

- Quality not quantity!

IMPORTANT

Be sure to use an anti-burst or burst resistant ball. The ball should be inflated well and should be firm.

EXERCISES ON THE BALL FOR BEGINNERS

If you have never used an exercise ball before try to familiarise yourself with basic movements. You can start to improve your core strength by simply sitting on it.

SWISS BALL EXERCISES

1 THE SEATED LEG RAISE

THE START POSITION

Sit on the ball with your feet flat on the floor in front of you and your arms relaxed by your sides. Raise one heel slowly to about knee height straightening your leg so it's parallel to the ground. Lower your leg and repeat on the other side.

Keeping your head up during the exercise will help you maintain your balance.

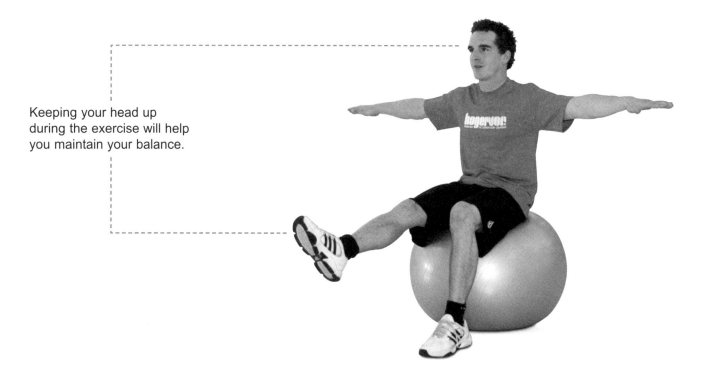

You can advance the movement by extending your arms sideways up to about shoulder level and/or holding your leg out straight for longer.

Repeat this for 10 reps.

IMPROVES BASIC BALANCE

2 BACK EXTENSIONS

THE START POSITION

Kneel on the floor facing the ball with your stomach and chest flat on the ball. Slowly extend your back lifting your chest off the ball. Your hands should be touching your ears and elbows pointing outwards. Squeeze your shoulder blades together as you lift off the ball.

Try to maintain a good body alignment throughout. Keep your breathing easy, relax your neck and keep your knees on the floor.

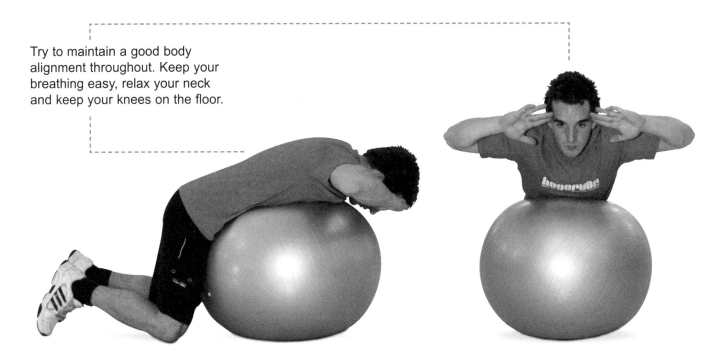

This exercise should be done in a slow controlled manner. Avoid doing this exercise if you suffer from any lower back pain.

Repeat this for 10 reps.

IMPROVES LOWER BACK STRENGTH

3 THE BALL PLANK - FOR CORE STRENGTH

THE START POSITION

Start by kneeling on the floor with your feet and shins resting on the ball behind you and your forearms flat on the floor. Slowly roll the ball backwards away from you, straightening your legs and supporting your weight on your forearms. Maintain a horizontal position parallel to the ground for as long as possible.

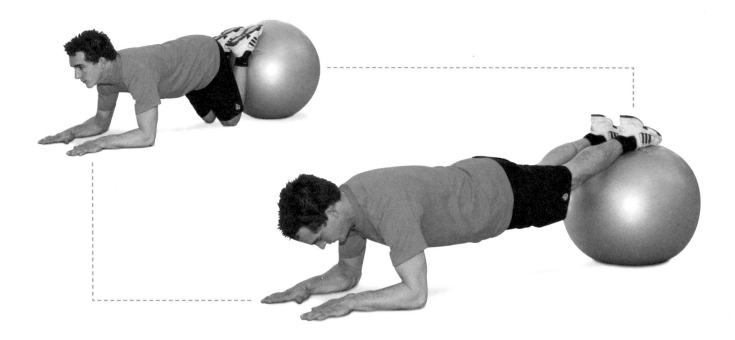

Keep your back straight while you are horizontal, squeeze your buttocks together and maintain tight abdominals throughout.

Repeat after a rest 3-4 times, recording your times to track your progression.

IMPROVES PADDLING STRENGTH

4 THE BALL PUSH-UP

THE START POSITION

Start by placing your feet on the ball supporting your weight on your hands in a press-up position. Keeping your back straight bend your elbows, slowly lowering your chest towards the floor. Slowly push back up, taking care to avoid locking your elbows at the top of the movement just before they fully extend.

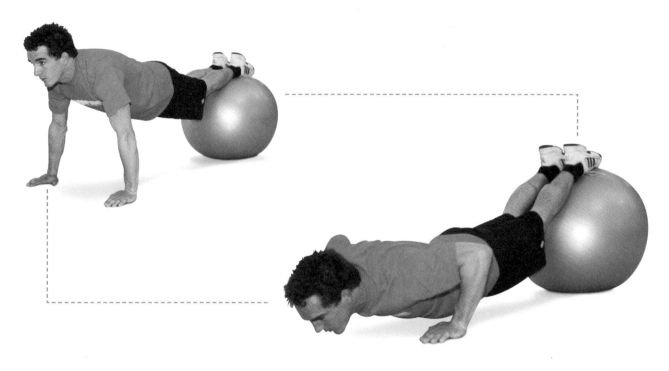

If you find this too wobbly then try to build up your core strength using the plank and basic press-ups first.

Repeat after a rest 3-4 times recording your times.

IMPROVES UPPER BODY STRENGTH

MOBILITY AND FLEXIBILITY USING THE BALL

The Swiss ball can be an excellent tool for improving a surfer's mobility and flexibility,
two very important factors in higher levels of surfing fitness.
Basic stretching keeps muscles in good form and supple, allowing the surfer to
push their range of surfing movements to greater heights. Remember to perform stretching
in a slow and controlled manner. Any sharp pain or overall discomfort should be avoided.

1 KNEELING BACK STRETCH

THE START POSITION

Sit backwards towards your heels. As you roll the ball forwards lengthen your torso from your hips to your fingers. You should feel the stretch through your arms, back and buttocks.

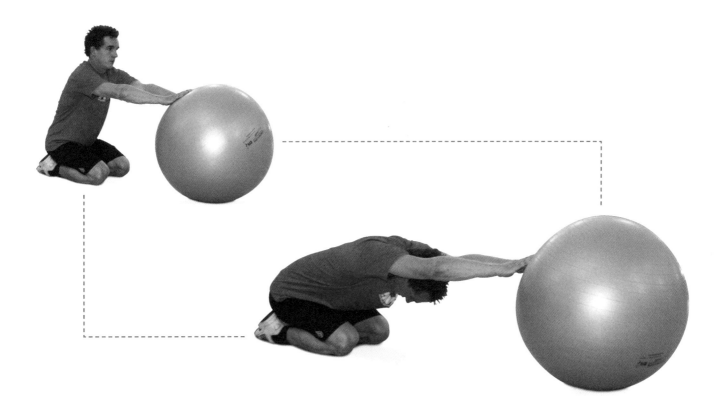

Hold each stretch for at least 10 seconds then roll back to the start position. Repeat 2-3 times.

IMPROVES PADDLING

2 CHEST STRETCH

THE START POSITION

Start by kneeling with the ball on your right hand side and your right hand and forearm resting on it. Lower your chest towards the floor supporting your body with your left hand. Look away from the ball as your lower your chest. You should feel a gentle stretch in front of your shoulder and across your chest.

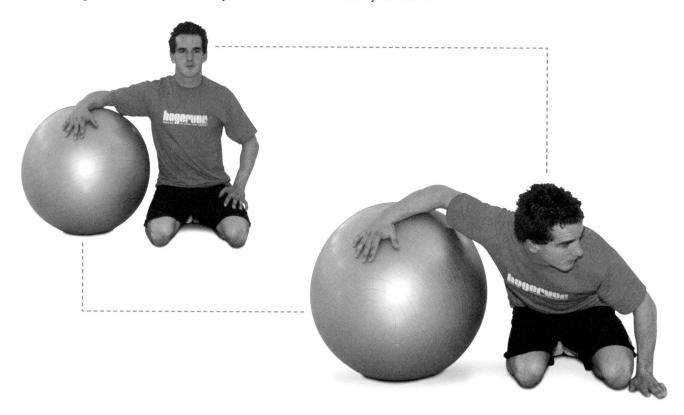

Hold the stretch for 10-15 seconds and then repeat on your left hand side.

STRETCHES THE PECTORALS

3 INNER THIGH STRENGTH

THE START POSITION

Start by sitting forward on the ball with your feet wide apart and your hands on your thighs. Roll slowly to your right side gradually straightening your left leg until you feel the stretch through your inner thigh.

Keeping your head up during the exercise will help you maintain your balance. Try to maintain a good body alignment throughout.

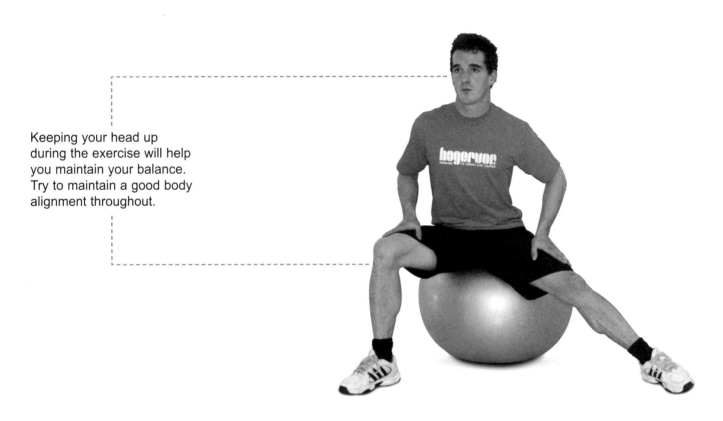

Hold for 15-20 seconds on the right and then repeat the same rolling to your left.

STRETCHES THE HIP FLEXOR

SWISS BALL EXERCISES

4 PRONE BACK STRETCH

THE START POSITION
Kneel on floor with the ball in front of you. Place your chest and arms on the ball and slowly raise your chest upwards extending your spine. You will only need to raise your chest a short distance to feel the stretch.

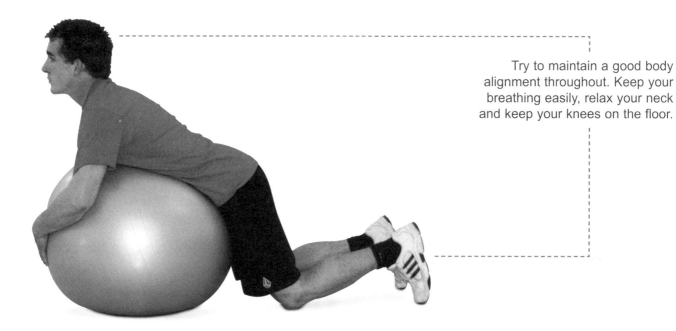

Try to maintain a good body alignment throughout. Keep your breathing easily, relax your neck and keep your knees on the floor.

Keep your knees and feet in contact with the floor throughout the movement and don't push yourself forwards whilst stretching.

Hold for 20 - 30 seconds and repeat 3 times.

AIDS INJURY PREVENTION

ROUND UP

These are just a few of the exercises available to the surfer to use as part of a training programme. The benefits are vast and open to all ages, from young groms just starting out to the well-seeded grandmaster. Swiss balls can be used in a warm-up session, cool-down session or in your main training set.

HOWEVER YOU DECIDE TO TRAIN WITH THE BALL, DON'T BLOW IT UP, ONLY USE IT ONCE AND THEN LEAVE IT COLLECTING DUST IN A CORNER SOMEWHERE!

SWISS BALL SIZES – CHOOSING A BALL

Due to the vast range of exercises available getting the right sized ball is vital. The cost of a Swiss ball will vary depending on size and quality.

CHOOSING A BALL   Make sure you use the right size ball for you

HEIGHT	BALL SIZE
IF YOU ARE LESS THAN 5'1"	45CM IN DIAMETER
IF YOU ARE 5'1" TO 5'8"	55CM IN DIAMETER
IF YOU ARE 5'8" TO 6'2"	65CM IN DIAMETER
IF YOU ARE OVER 6'	75CM IN DIAMETER

TOP TIP

THINGS TO REMEMBER

- Start off slowly and, as your strength increases, increase your speed.
- Maintain control and good posture throughout the exercise.
- Work hard on precision and not so much on speed.
- Quality not quantity!

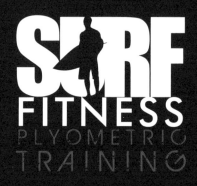

SURF
FITNESS
PLYOMETRIC
TRAINING

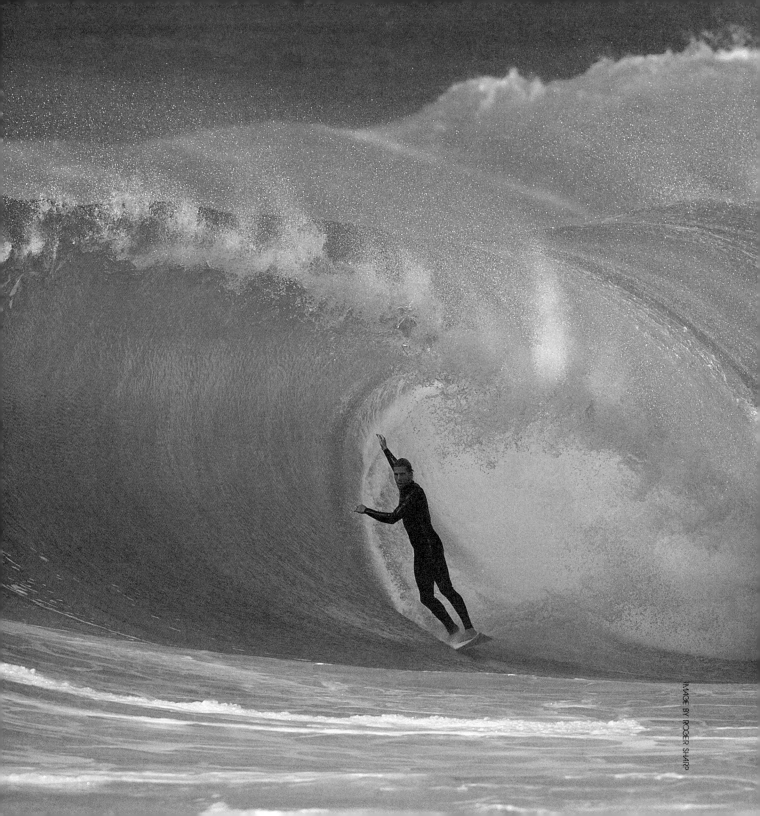

PLYOMETRIC

TRAINING

PLYOMETRICS
FOR EXPLOSIVE SURFING
POWER

WHAT IS PLYOMETRIC TRAINING?

Explosive speed and power are major components of your total surfing strength and are found in varying degrees in virtually all athletic movements. Over the years many sports coaches have used jumping and bouncing exercises to enhance athletic performance. This type of training in recent years has become known as plyometrics. Plyometrics is a term now used to describe any method of training that enhances your explosive movements.

By using high-quality and multi-directional drills, explosive movement and response times can be improved. Speed and agility are undoubtably highly desirable qualities in all surfing movements. Basic plyometric training in your training programme will sharpen your surfing movements making them faster.

Like many surfers, if you are not able to surf as often as you would like, explosive plyometric training will help keep you sharp while strengthening your body movements at the same time.

GETTING STARTED WITH THE BASICS

- It is very important to warm up before a plyometrics session with a light stretch.

- Avoid landing on your heels exercising on a hard surface, grass is ideal.

- Use only your body weight: all movements should be explosive with 100% effort.

- Avoid plyometric training two days in a row. Give yourself time to recover!

- A constant work rate is important, so make sure you rest for 60-90 seconds after each set.

- As your strength increases you can rest for a shorter period.

The benefits of plyometrics on surfing can be great. However they can be greatly reduced unless you train at least once a week and basic progression takes place. For major improvements in explosive power I recommend two or three 20-30 minute workouts a week as a good start.

1 ALTERNATING SQUAT THRUSTS INTO A SURFING POP UP

THE START POSITION

In a press-up position with your hands shoulder width apart, extend one leg back and the other leg forward towards your chest. Bring your extended leg forward and at the same time extend your bent leg, switching positions. Repeat this 6 times, then at speed move into a surfing pop-up, staying low for a split second. Then repeat your squat thrusts 6 times.

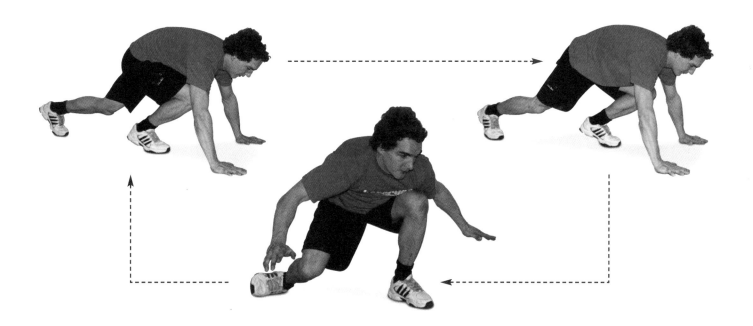

Keep this going for 30-40 seconds and complete 3-4 sets with 30 seconds rest after each. As you get fitter you can extend the length of time that you work for.

A QUICKER, MORE FLUID POP-UP

2 SQUAT THRUSTS INTO A SURFING POP-UP

THE START POSITION

In a press-up position with your hands shoulder width apart and both legs extended, bring your legs at speed towards your chest, then quickly extend them back. Repeat this motion 4 times then move into a surfing pop-up.

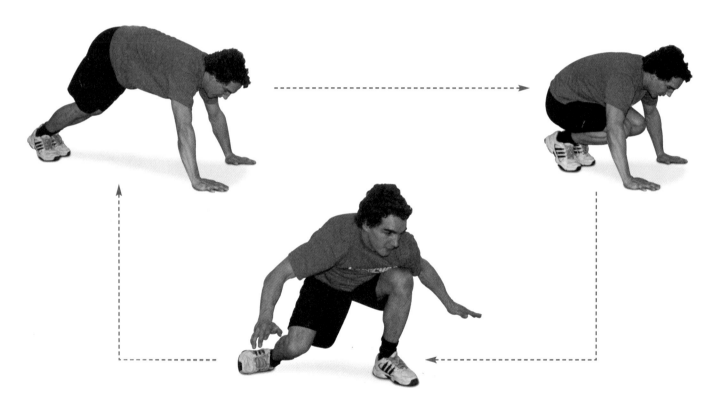

Keep this going for up to 60 seconds and complete 3-4 sets with 30 seconds rest after each. As you get fitter you can extend the length of time that you work for.

A QUICKER, MORE FLUID POP-UP

3 STANDING LONG JUMP

THE START POSITION

Start by standing with your feet together and your arms by your sides. Bend your knees and explode forwards using your arms to propel you forward. Try to land on the balls of your feet first.

Make sure you do this exercise on a suitable surface wearing appropriate footwear!

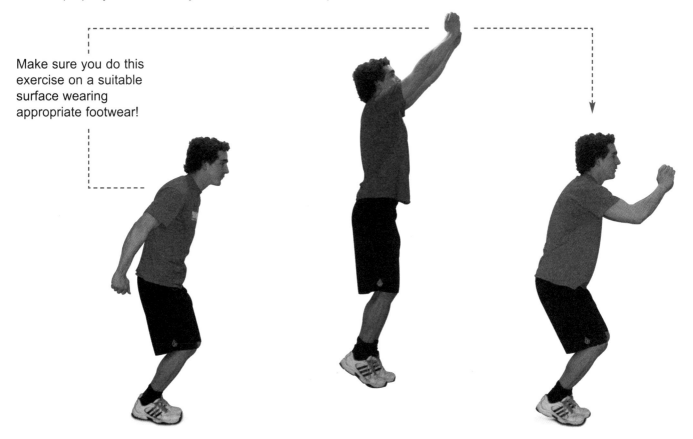

Do 10 jumps followed by 30 seconds rest and repeat 3-4 times.

INCREASES YOUR EXPLOSIVE POWER

4 LATERAL SIDE JUMPS

THE START POSITION
Stand on the left of a 20-25cm step. Jump from side to side across the step as fast as you can. Keep your feet together and stay in control of the movement at all times. Make sure when jumping you stay on the balls of your feet.

Please make sure you do this exercise on a suitable surface wearing appropriate footwear!

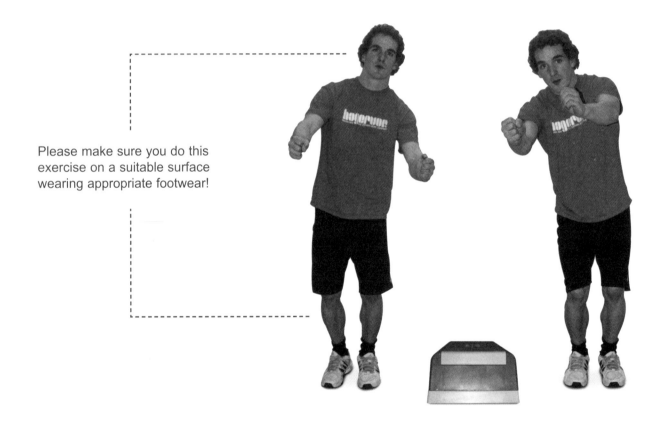

Do 10 jumps followed by 30 seconds rest. Repeat the set of 10, 3-4 times.

INCREASES YOUR EXPLOSIVE POWER

5 THE BOX JUMP

THE START POSITION

Find a sturdy box or step about 30cm in height. Stand with the box in front of you, your feet together and your arms by your sides. Jump onto the box using as much explosive power as possible. Again try to land on the balls of your feet.

Please make sure whatever you are jumping onto is on a suitable non-slip surface

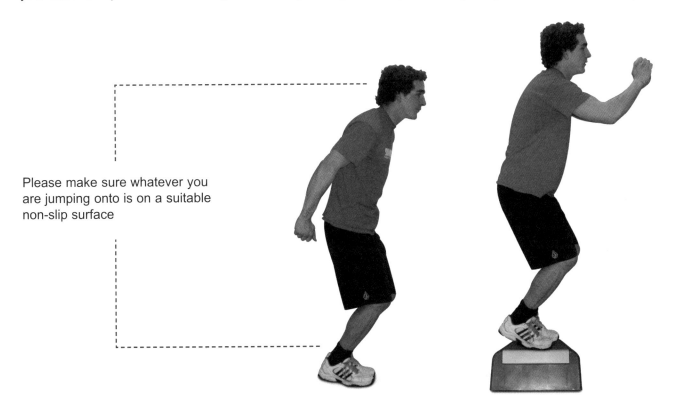

MAKE SURE THE BOX IS ON A LEVEL FLOOR AND IS NOT GOING TO MOVE WHEN YOU JUMP ONTO IT!

Do 10 jumps followed by 30 seconds rest and repeat 3-4 times. As you improve gradually increase the height of the box.

INCREASES YOUR EXPLOSIVE POWER

PLYOMETRIC TRAINING

6 VERTICAL JUMPS

THE START POSITION
Start by standing with your feet together and your arms by your sides.
Bend your knees and explode upwards as far as you can with your
arms extended.

Try to land on the balls of your feet and bend your knees to absorb the impact.

It might sound obvious, but
check the height of the ceiling
before you start jumping!

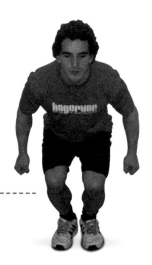

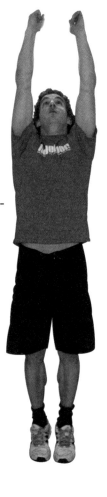

Do 10 jumps followed by 30-45 seconds rest and repeat 3-4 times.

INCREASES YOUR EXPLOSIVE POWER

PLYOMETRIC WORKOUT

I RECOMMEND 2-3 20-30 MINUTE WORKOUTS A WEEK

As always, a comprehensive warm-up is important before you start, along with some light mobility exercises

WARM-UP
Start with a gentle 8-10 minute run. During your run add a few heel taps and knee lifts to improve the effectiveness of your warm-up.

Follow your run with 5/6 minutes of very basic stretches. Once you've finished stretching, you are ready to start.

SUGGESTED WORKOUT
--->

- 3 sets of 10 box jumps.
- 3 sets of 10 side jumps (lateral side jumps).
- 3 sets of 10 vertical jumps.
- 3 sets of 10 squat thrusts into a surfing pop-up.

After each set of 10 take 30 seconds rest. For basic progression just add an extra few jumps to each workout. Take a 4-5 minute rest after each exercise.

TOP TIP

ALTERNATIVE PLYOMETRICS SESSIONS
If you want to vary your workout, an alternative plyometrics session for improving your surfing explosive power could be low hurdle jumps or advanced bounding and hopping.

IMPORTANT TO REMEMBER
If you suffer from any knee or hip problems, you should avoid plyometrics due to the repeated explosive movements involved.

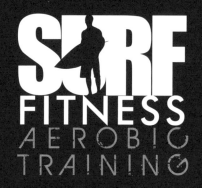

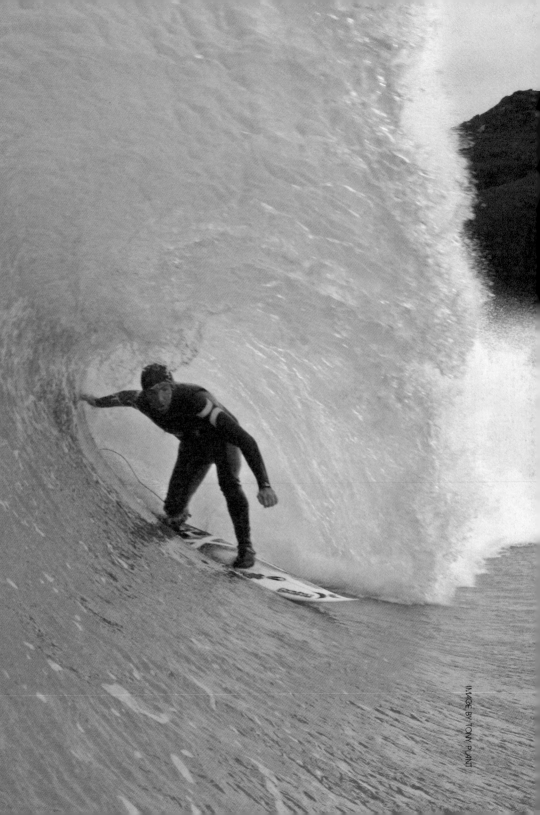

WHAT IS AEROBIC TRAINING?

Aerobic literally means "with air". As a surfer it is extremely beneficial to build up aerobic fitness. This can be achieved through a wide range of training and is known as an aerobic base.

Selecting the type of aerobic exercise that you engage in should be done with surfing in mind.

AEROBIC
TRAINING

AEROBIC TRAINING FOR SURF FITNESS

Generally speaking it would be best to combine both swimming and running in your aerobic training programme – this is known as cross training. Raising the level of aerobic training that you do i.e. anaerobic (without oxygen) training will also help to boost your fitness levels.

If you are seriously de-conditioned or have current problems with your knees, back or similar, it may be wise to avoid high-impact aerobic training like running to start with and stick to swimming.

You can measure aerobic intensity in three different ways, but using your heart rate is the most precise method. This is most effectively done using a portable heart rate monitor which can be purchased almost everywhere these days.

HOW LONG SHOULD YOU TRAIN TO IMPROVE AEROBIC FITNESS?

The length of time that you train for aerobically will depend on your surfing goals. If you are a competing surfer or surf on a very regular basis, you may wish to aim for top aerobic fitness levels. Generally speaking, 40-60 minutes of moderate aerobic training 2-4 times per week will dramatically increase your aerobic fitness.

WHAT TYPES OF AEROBIC INTENSITIES ARE THERE?

Aerobic levels can be measured by using a heart rate monitoring system. As a guide to your maximum heart rate (MHR), subtract your age in years from 220 for a male and from 226 for a female. Resting and maximum heart rates are influenced by activity and age. As a result of higher levels of activity and increased fitness your resting heart rate will decrease.

If you are to boost your levels of aerobic fitness then it is important that you work at different percentage rates of your MHR.For example, if you were to train at a chilled out 60-70% of your MHR, your levels of fitness will remain low. This can be termed as low-end aerobic activity. Studies have shown that training must exceed a certain minimum threshold if significant changes in aerobic fitness are to occur.

FINDING YOUR MAXIMUM HEART RATE

As an example, a 25 year old man using the MHR formula (220-25) will have an MHR of 195. Working at 65-75% of 195 would be considered low-end aerobic training. Depending on your fitness levels this type of aerobic training is relatively stress free.

If you are looking to boost your aerobic fitness to higher levels then working out at around 80-85% of your MHR is a must. Working at higher levels of aerobic training is much more demanding, and training at this level will require a much shorter training time as air will be in much shorter supply.

If you are working out at a low-end aerobic level then holding a conversation during exercise should not be a problem. Working out at a high-end aerobic level will leave you out of breath and only able to talk for a short length of time.

EXAMPLES OF LOW-END AEROBIC TRAINING

A slow steady jog or swim for around 40-50 minutes will not boost your aerobic fitness to superman levels but it will play a major role in building a good aerobic fitness base. Due to the low impact of low-end aerobic training on the body's energy levels, this type of training can be done 3-5 times a week. Try to break this regime up with some sort of recovery phase, i.e. one day on, one day off. If you are just starting out on a new fitness programme or are returning to exercise from a long lay off, then this is a good type of training for you. It will allow your body to ease into things and will reduce the risk of injury.

EXAMPLES OF HIGH-END INTERVAL TRAINING

A good example of high-end aerobic exercise would be 2 x 10 minute runs with a rest period of around 2 minutes walking or at a slow steady jog to recover. If you are training on a regular basis then your ability to do more high-end work should improve, providing your training programme is progressive and constructive. During this type of training you should aim to be working at 80-85% of your MHR.

AEROBIC TRAINING

A BASIC AEROBIC FITNESS PROGRAMME – WEEK BY WEEK

WEEKS 1-2	1-2 steady jogs at 65-75% of your MHR	A gradual progression in the intensity of your programme will ensure that your sessions are constructive
WEEKS 3-4	1-2 steady jogs at 65-75% of your MHR and 6-8 min run at 80-85% of your MHR	
WEEKS 5-6	1-3 steady jogs at 65-75% of your MHR and 8-12 min run at 80-85% of your MHR	
WEEKS 7-8	2-3 steady jogs at 65-75% of your MHR and 2 x 8 min runs at 80-85% of your MHR with 90 sec steady jog as a recovery	

You may wish to start with short jogs i.e. 20-30 mins then build up your distance as you begin to feel stronger. Try to make a record of your distance, time and amount of heart rate work that you do.

ANAEROBIC TRAINING - WITHOUT OXYGEN

Anaerobic training is much shorter in its duration than aerobic training. Working at levels of heart rate just outside the high-end aerobic (85%+) will limit your oxygen levels even further. As a surfer, anaerobic training can be extremely useful.

Depending on the break you surf, where in the world and the conditions at the time you paddle out, you can be left breathless and a bit worn out. Most surfers paddling out through 2-3ft surf and upwards have at some point put in a reasonable amount of effort to get out back. Your heart rate will rise and depending on the length of the paddle, may well reach 80-95% of your MHR. Some form of anaerobic training each week can boost your paddle power, leaving you fresher and ready for your first set instead of sitting on your board for 10 minutes wondering why it took you so long!

High levels of anaerobic training in general will last no longer than 2 minutes per effort. Constructing some form of programme either in the gym, out running or in the pool in the form of intervals is the best form of anaerobic training.

BASIC ANAEROBIC TRAINING SETS

Anaerobic training can be a very stressful type of training. A basic level of fitness is needed before undertaking high levels of anaerobic training. Make sure you follow a good warm-up procedure before any anaerobic training. Avoid intense anaerobic training sessions two days in a row.

RUNNING AS AN ANAEROBIC EXERCISE

After 10-15 minutes running at a moderate pace, aim to run at a target HR of between 85-95% over short bursts of about 60-90 seconds.

Depending on your fitness levels you should start with 4-6 reps of 60-90 second runs at your target HR with a rest period of 30-40 seconds between each set.

As your fitness improves, you will be able to increase the amount of runs per week using anaerobic training by 1-2 sessions. Even one session of anaerobic training a week will be a great boost to your general surfing fitness.

For anaerobic training in the pool check out the swim training section.

TOP TIP

NEW TO TRAINING?

If you are new to training, light aerobic training for several weeks is advisable. Using a heart rate monitoring system will be of great benefit to any training surfer.

Always make sure you follow a good warm-up and cool-down programme for injury prevention.

As a surfer it is extremely beneficial to build up aerobic fitness.

Selecting the type of aerobic exercise that you engage in should be done with surfing in mind.

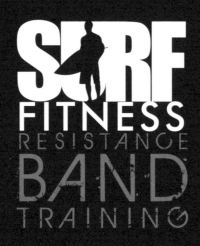

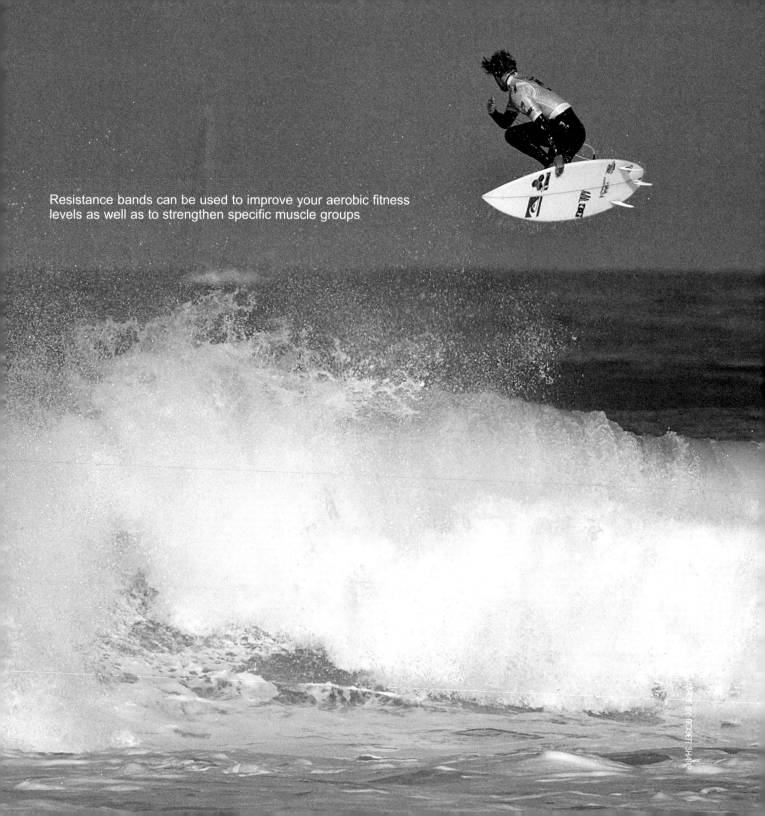

Resistance bands can be used to improve your aerobic fitness
levels as well as to strengthen specific muscle groups

IMAGE BY ROGER SHARP

RESISTANCE BAND
TRAINING

WHAT IS RESISTANCE BAND TRAINING?

Resistance bands are used as a training aid across the world. They have a whole range of uses, from general strength and conditioning to rehabilitation or injury prevention.

Resistance band exercises are ideal for surfing fitness as they improve strength for paddling and aid injury prevention. Resistance bands can also be used to improve your aerobic fitness levels when incorporated into a circuit training format as well as to strengthen specific muscle groups. Resistance bands will strengthen and elongate your muscle fibres, stimulating growth and improving your full range of movement. Keep your resistance band exercises progressive. Increase the number of reps in each exercise as your strength increases.

Unlike free weights, resistance bands provide the surfer with constant tension on the muscles. The band allows you to focus on the concentric (lifting) portion and the eccentric (lowering) portion of any movement.

If you are thinking of starting a resistance band training programme, then good-quality resistance bands with handles are best.

GETTING STARTED

As with any workout, make sure you warm up properly before. Your workout should include a full range of body movements.

Resistance bands are available in a range of colours; these often relate to their overall resistance. A surfer seeking to improve strength and endurance will need at least 3-4 bands of differing resistance levels.

WHAT ARE THE BENEFITS?

These 5 exercises will aid and improve your upper body surfing strength. As with any exercise programme it is advisable to work all major muscle groups in a balanced programme for total body conditioning. Add these exercises to your weekly programme and always follow the basic workout format, i.e. warm up and cool down.

As a surfer wishing to improve your endurance, try boosting your reps to as many as 30 over a 5-6 week training phase or go for duration i.e. 60 seconds non-stop over 3-4 sets.

WHAT YOU CAN HOPE TO ACHIEVE

The goal of resistance band training is to gradually and progressively overload the musculoskeletal system so it gets stronger. Research shows that regular training with resistance bands will strengthen and tone muscles.

Resistance band training is a form of training in which each effort is performed against a specific opposing force generated by resistance, i.e. pushed, stretched or bent. Exercises are isotonic if a body part is moving against a force. Exercises are isometric if a body part is holding still against a force.

TOP TIP

WHAT MAKES RESISTANCE BANDS A MUST HAVE?

Resistance bands are an often overlooked piece of training equipment. Their portability and endless range of exercises make them the perfect training aid for surfers.

1 REVERSE FLYE

Trapezius and back of shoulders.

THE START POSITION

Stand on the centre of the band holding the handles in front of you with your feet together. Lean forwards bending at the waist with soft knees. Bend your elbows slightly and extend your arms out to the side bringing your hands up level with your chest. Squeeze your back as you do so.

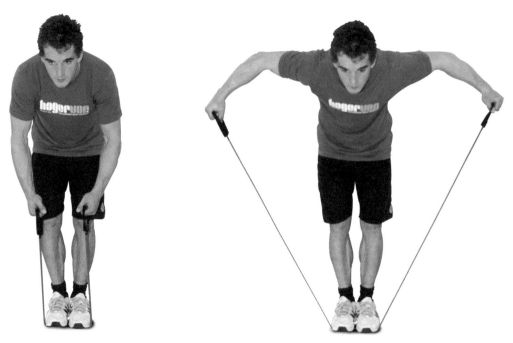

Make sure that you use the right band for the exercise. The band needs to provide enough resistance for it to be effective, but it should not be so tight it's uncomfortable to fully extend it.

Repeat this for 12-15 reps.

IMPROVES PADDLE STRENGTH

2 CHEST PRESS
Pectorals.

THE START POSITION
Wrap the resistance band around something stable behind you and take a handle in each hand. The band should be running along the inside of your forearms and your hands should be level with your chest. Slowly press your arms out in front of you level with your chest.

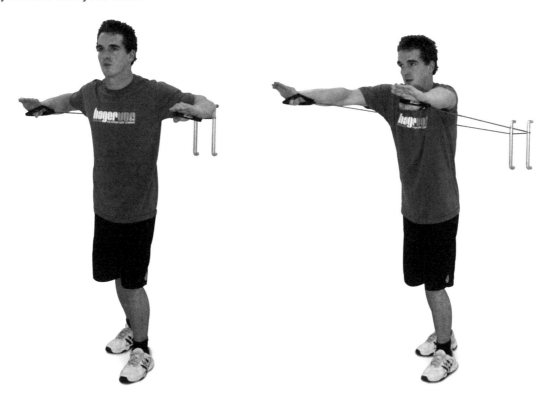

To increase the resistance of the exercise step forwards stretching the band.

Repeat this for 12-15 reps.

IMPROVES POP-UPS AND PADDLE STRENGTH

3 SINGLE ARM LATERAL RAISE
Deltoids.

THE START POSITION
Stand with one end of the band under your right foot and the other in your left hand. Keeping your elbow slightly bent lift your arm out to your left hand side to shoulder level then slowly back to the start position.

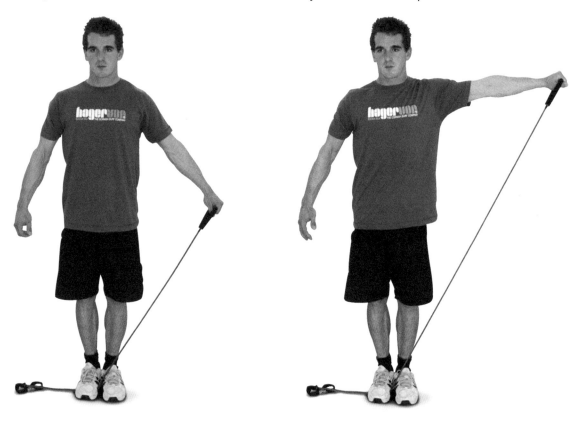

Repeat this for 12-15 reps on your left arm then switch and repeat on your right.

IMPROVES PADDLE STRENGTH

4 TRICEP EXTENSIONS

THE START POSITION

Stand with your legs hip width apart. Grasp the band with your left hand behind your back at waist height and with your right hand behind your head over your right shoulder. Keeping your left arm locked in position, extend your right arm upwards taking care not to lock your right arm out fully.

It's important to maintain a good body alignment throughout the exercise

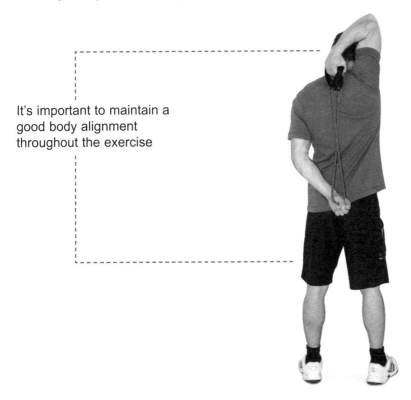
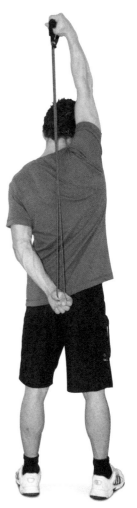

Repeat this for 12-15 reps on your right arm then switch and repeat on your left arm.

IMPROVES PADDLE STRENGTH

5 SEATED ROW

THE START POSITION

Place the band around a step, or another suitable, stable piece of equipment. Lean back to tension the band and raise your arms horizontally in front of you. Once you have moderate tension pull your elbows backwards bringing your hands towards your chest and squeeze your shoulder blades together.

Keep your head up
and your back straight
throughout the exercises

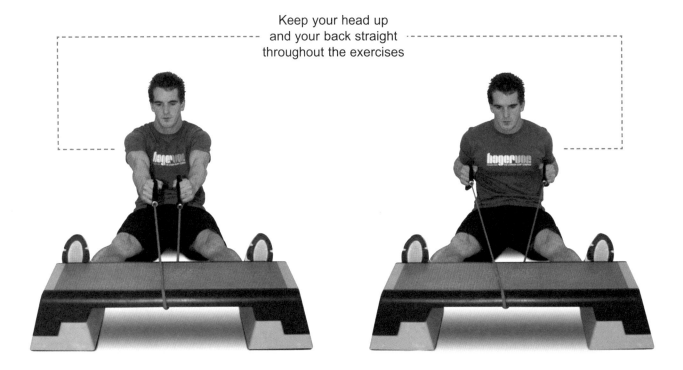

If you don't have a step or any other suitable equipment, you can wrap the bands around your feet.

Repeat this for 12-15 reps to start. Increase reps as your strength improves.

IMPROVES PADDLE STRENGTH & YOUR POP-UP POWER

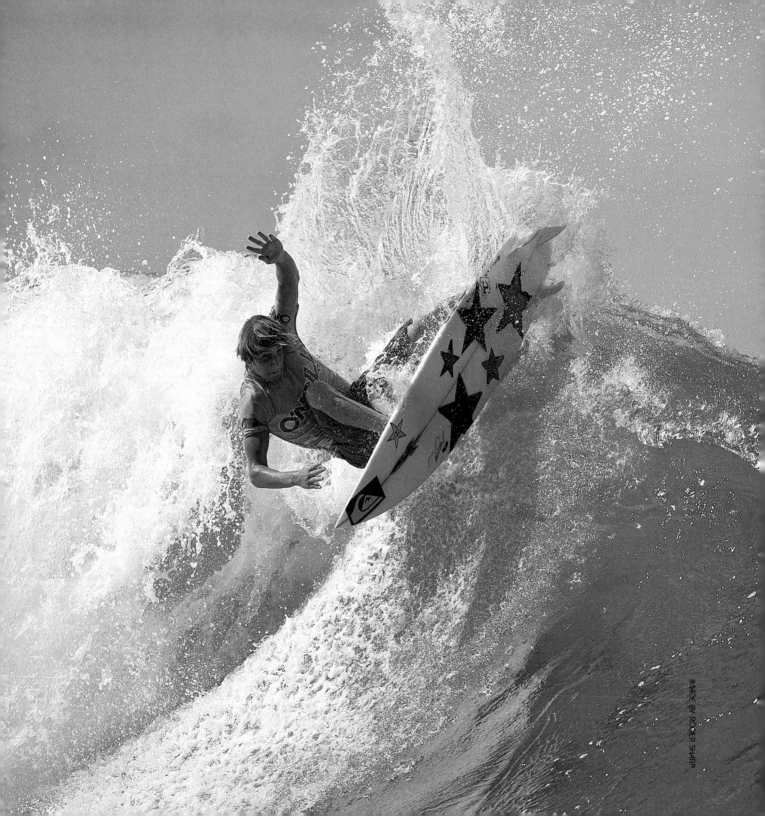

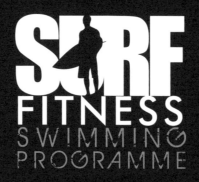

SURF
FITNESS
SWIMMING
PROGRAMME

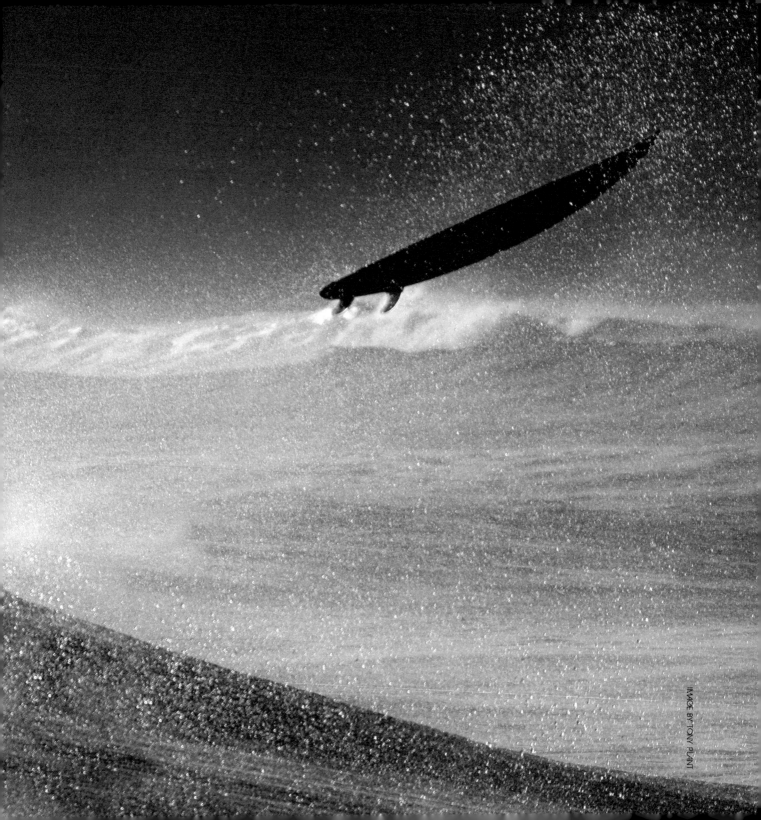

SWIMMING

PROGRAMMES

BASIC SWIMMING PROGRAMMES FOR SURFING STRENGTH

As a surfer, swimming has to be one of the best ways to improve your surfing fitness. Swimming 2-3 times a week can make a massive difference to your paddle power.

If you are a regular swimmer, or intend to become one, but you are unable to swim basic front crawl, then learning front crawl or improving your stroke will help you to increase your fitness levels more efficiently. If you feel that your swimming technique is not up to much and needs improvement then contact a local swimming coach for some help. A good technique will not only improve your training session but will also reduce your risk of injury through poor technique.

Jumping in the pool each week and swimming a set distance each time will be of some benefit to your surfing, but a planned weekly programme of swimming will help you boost your fitness levels dramatically.

TYPES OF SWIMMING TRAINING FOR SURFING FITNESS

Low-end aerobic swimming will help you increase your swimming strength slowly but surely. If you are looking to start a constructive swimming programme for the first time you should swim at a steady pace, about 60-70% of your MHR for 30-40 minutes 2-3 times a week for 4-6 weeks. Once you have built up a good base and your fitness levels have risen, then it's a good time to start thinking about some basic swimming programmes.

TYPES OF PADDLE FITNESS

CHILLED-OUT PADDLE SPEED
Low end aerobic
60-70% of your MHR

INTERMEDIATE PADDLE SPEED
Mid to high-end aerobic
75-85% of your MHR

SUPER FAST PADDLE SPEED
Anaerobic 85-95% of your MHR

With all these types of fitness levels taking place during just one surf, it's wise to boost your swimming fitness to accommodate all three!

WARMING UP FOR A SWIMMING SESSION

As with all of your workouts it's essential you follow a comprehensive warm-up procedure before your session.

SLOW MOBILISATION OF ALL LIMBS AND JOINTS
This will increase blood flow to all working muscles and help warm up your body temperature.

A LIGHT ALL OVER BODY STRETCH,
Holding each stretch for around 8-10 seconds.

A LIGHT SWIM
This should be done without pause and should last (depending on ability) for around 10-12 minutes.

EXAMPLE WARM UP
500m swim with each 100m getting faster by about 10%. Or start at a very low impact aerobic swimming level progressing to a high-end aerobic swim.

SWIMMING EQUIPMENT

There are several pieces of equipment available to you that will help improve your surfing and swimming strength.

THE SWIM PULLBUOY
A great tool for improving general upper body strength. Placed between your legs, it keeps your lower body buoyant allowing you to pull through the water using only your upper body.

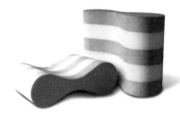

EXTRA LARGE RESISTANCE BANDS
These can be used for whole workouts if you can't get to the pool. They can be used to mimic most swimming movements by fixing them to a solid base. They're a great bit of kit and you don't even need to get your hair wet!

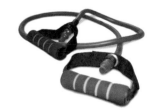

SWIMMING PROGRAMMES

BASIC SWIMMING PROGRAMMES - FOR SURFING STRENGTH

The swimming distances in these programmes can be adjusted depending on your ability. If you are just starting out then start swimming short distances and slowly build up your distance as your swimming improves.

Even a basic swimming programme should be progressive. Keep a record of your target times and distances including your warm-up and cool-down sessions.

BASIC SWIMMING TRAINING
Light aerobic

WARM UP	MAIN SESSION	COOL OFF
Basic mobility 4 - 5 mins Gentle stretch 4 - 5 mins Hold each for 8 - 10 secs	Swim 12 x 50m front crawl with 5 - 10 secs rest after each 50m Breathing should be relaxed	Swim 300 - 400m slow and easy with each consecutive lap getting slower
Swim non stop for 300 - 400m front crawl with each consecutive length getting faster	1 x 400m front crawl at the same pace with a pull float	Stretch for 6 - 8 mins covering all major muscle groups. Hold each stretch for 15 - 20 secs

As your swimming fitness improves you will find that you are able to maintain a lower heart rate for your main session set of 12 x 50m with 10 secs rest. Initially it may be beneficial to take a longer rest period if you are not a strong swimmer.

Once you are able to do a basic distance like 400m without stopping, you may wish to add an extra 400m, i.e. 2 x 400m with a rest interval of 60 secs.

If your swimming fitness is very basic you will find that your heart rate will go above the low-end aerobic level during longer swims (50m+), it may even reach high-end aerobic levels and above. This is normal but with regular training you will find it much easier to maintain a low heart rate.

BASIC SWIMMING TRAINING
Anaerobic

TARGET HR – 85-95% OF YOUR MHR

WARM UP	MAIN SESSION	COOL OFF
Basic mobility 4 - 5 mins Gentle stretch 4 - 5 mins Hold each for 8 - 10 secs	Swim 3 x 100m front crawl with 30 secs rest after each 100m Check your HR	Swim 500m slow and easy with each consecutive lap getting slower
Swim non stop for 400m+ front crawl with each consecutive lap getting faster	2 x 150m front crawl with 45 secs rest after each 150m Check your HR	Stretch for 8 - 10 mins covering all major muscle groups. Hold each stretch for 15 - 20 secs

You may wish to add a slow, low-end aerobic swim using a pull float to your main session of around 300 – 500m

The distances in this basic swimming programme will not be suitable for all abilities. You may wish to reduce your time period and increase distance and reps. Once your ability improves, your swimming will become much more manageable.

BASIC KICK SET

If you are able to complete basic swimming training on a regular weekly basis then kicking sets will be of great benefit for developing and maintaining your technique. A good kick adds balance to your stroke and aids propulsion.

Holding a float with your arms extended swim 4 x 25m with 10 seconds rest between each. Repeat this 2-3 times with an additional rest after each set of 4.

If you're already a competent swimmer then try kicking 50m-400m with a little longer rest. You can increase the kicking distance according to your level of ability. If you've got a poor kick this could be down to foot position and ankle flexibility; try kicking with fins on.

SWIMMING PROGRAMMES

BASIC SPRINT SET

Swimming training at full speed i.e. 100% effort, 95-100% of your MHR can be of great benefit to any surfer. Whether you are paddling to make a sneaky set or finding yourself on a fat one, sprint training can help you.

Sprint training in the pool should be kept to a minimum; sprinting every day in the pool is not advisable. Add small amounts to your swim training programme for best results, making sure to warm up before you do so. Try to stick to front crawl for your sprint training as this stroke is the most similar movement to paddling.

SPRINT SET BREAKDOWN

- Big warm up, at least a steady 10 minute swim.

- Swim 4 x 25m front crawl flat out with 60 seconds rest between each 25m.

- Swim 4 x 25m front crawl but only sprint half a length with 30 secs rest between each 25m.

- Swim 4 x 25m front crawl. Towards the end of each length you should swim progressively faster.

PROGRESSING THE EXERCISE

After 2-3 weeks you may wish to progress your sprint set.

ADD AN EXTRA 25-50M ON THE SETS EACH WEEK.

TOP TIP

BASIC SPRINT TRAINING
- A good warm up is highly advisable.
- Give yourself a week's break from sprinting every 4 weeks for recovery.
- Give yourself a good swim cool-down after sprint sets to aid recovery.

SWIMMING FITNESS TESTS

If you are training in the pool for additional surfing fitness it may be beneficial to record the results from your training sessions in a weekly diary. In addition to this you may wish to test your swimming fitness levels with a swimming fitness test. Fitness tests are a great way to monitor fitness levels and can be done at almost any time during a fitness programme.

Listed below are two basic swimming fitness tests. As with any intense exercise, your warm-up becomes even more important. A constructive warm-up with mobility stretches will aid the test results. Once the test is over a cool-down period is also advisable as this will aid recovery

TEST 1 – THE TT OR TIME TRIAL

This is basically a distance swim over a set time.
E.g. Swim as far as you can in 20 minutes then record the distance.

TEST 2 – THE BASIC HR TEST OR HEART RATE TEST

There are many different types of HR tests available. For the most accurate reading use a Heart Rate Monitor.

After warming up swim a short set distance e.g. 200m as fast as you can at 100% effort. As soon as you finish take your HR. Continue to record your HR at set timed periods to track the progress of the improvements in your recovery rate.

EXAMPLE HEART RATE TEST

- Immediately after exercise – record HR

- 30 seconds after exercise – record HR

- 60 seconds after exercise – record HR

Keep a record of all four resting HR and repeat every four weeks. As you get fitter your HR readings should fall and you should recover faster.

ALWAYS USE THE SAME DISTANCE AND COOL-DOWN FOR EACH TEST

SWIMMING PROGRAMMES

HYPOXIC SWIMMING TRAINING – BREATH HOLDING

As surfers we have all been there, that hold-down after getting nailed by a wave, that feeling that you're not coming up and fast running out of air! A feeling made much worse by the fact that you are being rolled around underwater like a rag doll. Over the years there have been many suggestions on how to deal with a major hold-down or wipeout. The plain fact is there really is no perfect way to train for it! Inevitably in this situation your movements become faster and more desperate the longer you are under. This increase in speed of movement will use up what oxygen you have left in your body even faster, causing you to panic even more.

Many surfers say they try to relax during a long hold-down, which is what we should all do in an ideal world. Your heart rate is slower when you are relaxed, thus your demand for oxygen decreases. Actually putting this technique into practice can be easier said than done. A more practical solution is to increase your lung capacity. This will enable you to take on increased levels of oxygen and give you valuable extra seconds under water. Breath holding in a pool can help you prepare for this unavoidable situation and is known as hypoxic (low oxygen) swimming training.

HYPOXIC TRAINING FOR THAT LONG HOLD-DOWN

Hypoxic (low oxygen) training was developed some years ago and can significantly help swimmers to maintain a smooth stroke when the pressure is on over a set racing distance. Or in your case, help make the inevitable hold down less daunting.

BASIC HYPOXIC TRAINING PROGRAMME

- Warm up, at least a steady 10 minute swim.

- Swim 4 x 50m front crawl breathing every 4 strokes with 30 secs rest after each 50m.
  Take 60 secs rest after the last 50m.

- Swim 2 x 100m front crawl breathing every 5 strokes with 60 secs rest aftereach 100m.
  Take 60 secs rest after the last 100m.

- Finish the set with 4 x 25m front crawl, breathing once mid-length.

THIS BASIC PROGRAMME WILL NOT BE SUITABLE FOR EVERYONE AND CAN BE TAILORED TO SUIT YOUR LEVEL OF ABILITY. IF YOU SUFFER FROM RESPIRATORY PROBLEMS LIKE ASTHMA THEN EXTRA CARE SHOULD BE TAKEN.

EXAMPLE OF A WEEKLY HYPOXIC TRAINING SET

If you are new to swimming then extra care should be taken with any breath holding exercises.

SWIMMING PROGRAMME 1- 2 TIMES PER WEEK

Warm up as normal before starting, as you should before any swimming session. This example swimming programme consists of 2 sets of 12 x 25m front crawl, which should initially be swum at a steady pace that you are comfortable with. After each 25m take 30 secs rest. If you're a regular swimmer the rest interval may need adjusting. After each 12 x 25m you may wish to take several minutes rest to recover.

Each week reduce the number of breaths you take per length. As you get better at holding your breath you may wish to increase the distance you swim.

Once you have adapted to breath holding you may wish to increase the speed at which you swim from a steady to a moderate pace.

5 WEEK HYPOXIC TRAINING PROGRAMME

WEEK	WEEK 1	WEEK 2	WEEK 3	WEEK 4	WEEK 5
SWIM SET BREAKDOWN	2 sets 12 x 25m front crawl 60 secs rest after each 12 10 secs after each 25m	2 sets 12 x 25m front crawl 60 secs rest after each 12 10 secs after each 25m	2 sets 12 x 25m front crawl 60 secs rest after each 12 10 secs after each 25m	2 sets 12 x 25m front crawl 60 secs rest after each 12 10 secs after each 25m	2 sets 12 x 25m front crawl 60 secs rest after each 12 10 secs after each 25m
BREATHING RATE	EVERY 4 STROKES	EVERY 5 STROKES	EVERY 6 STROKES	EVERY 7 STROKES	EVERY 8 STROKES

A good way to test your progress during a hypoxic training programme is to swim as far as you can underwater every six weeks and record the distance.

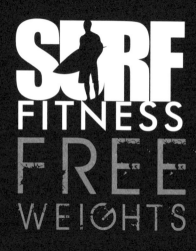

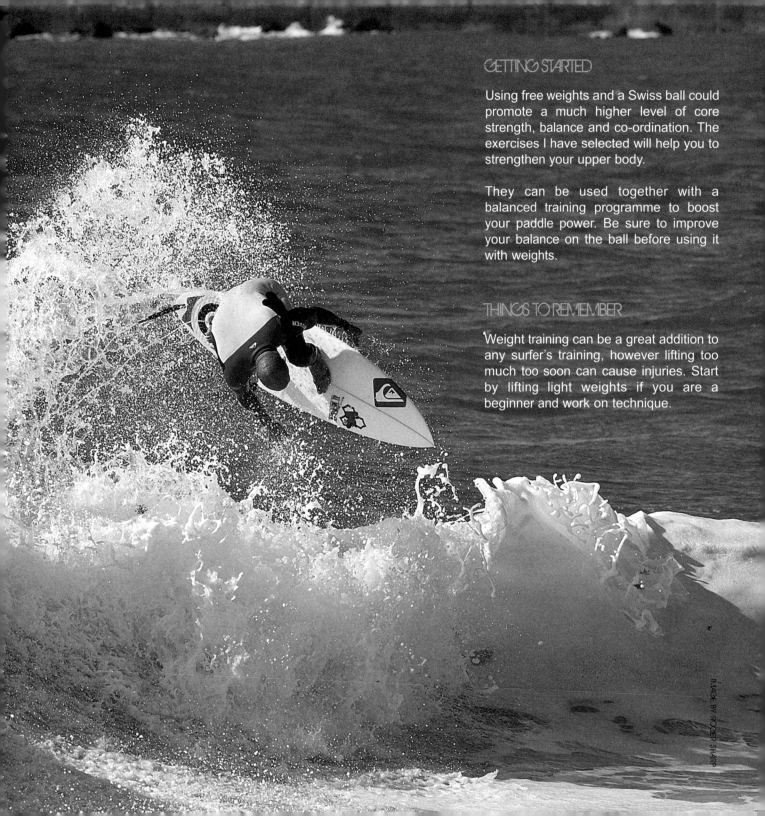

GETTING STARTED

Using free weights and a Swiss ball could promote a much higher level of core strength, balance and co-ordination. The exercises I have selected will help you to strengthen your upper body.

They can be used together with a balanced training programme to boost your paddle power. Be sure to improve your balance on the ball before using it with weights.

THINGS TO REMEMBER

Weight training can be a great addition to any surfer's training, however lifting too much too soon can cause injuries. Start by lifting light weights if you are a beginner and work on technique.

IMAGE BY ROGER SHARP

FREE WEIGHTS

FREE WEIGHTS - FOR SURFING STRENGTH

A basic free weights programme can make all the difference to a surfer's strength and endurance. As with all sports, just any old exercise programme is not going to help you achieve the best possible results.

Sport specific training is the best way to train for any sport. A tailored weights programme with surfing movements in mind i.e. paddle power, will be of most benefit to you. With any resistance training you should follow an all over, well-balanced programme which covers all the major muscle groups.

As a surfer it is important to remember that maintaining a good range of movement is vital. This should be reflected in your weight training programme. Lifting heavy weights time after time could restrict a surfer's range of movement, leaving you slow and sluggish. Combining a light to medium weight, high rep workout with a good flexibility programme could well be the best option.

STAY INJURY FREE WHEN LIFTING WEIGHTS

ALWAYS WARM UP

Warming up will minimize your risk of injury. It will prepare your body for your workout and increase blood flow to the working muscles. Mobility exercises and an 8-10 minute cardio warm up will increase your heart rate slowly.

GOOD TECHNIQUE

Always use weights with a good technique in mind. This is a must and will reduce your risk of injury. It will also reduce the amount of stress on your joints and ligaments. Seek professional advice if you are not sure how to lift weights correctly. All lifting should be done without jerky movements and with a good posture.

Resist the extra 2 reps if your technique has failed. You need to overload your muscles but not to the point of injury.

THE PROS & CONS OF FREE WEIGHTS AGAINST MACHINES

If you are a regular gym user you'll more than likely at some point have thought, which is better, free weights or machines? Each can be of benefit but there are definite differences in both. If you are just starting out on a new weight programme then machines may well be the better route. They offer a safer option to that of weights with regards to technique.

There has been research undertaken which has shown that using free weights could promote quicker strength gains as well as improving your balance and co-ordination. By lifting free weights you will use more core strength during movements and recruit more muscle groups than machines are able to.

As a surfer training for additional fitness, the range of movement and core strength should be of high priority. You may wish to adopt a free weights and machine workout, but long-term free weights for surfing strength could well be the better option.

FOLLOW A WEIGHTS ROUTINE THAT IS RIGHT FOR SURFING

EXAMPLE 1
Adopt a training programme that increases your rep count as you get stronger. One form of progression could be to add an extra 2-3 reps to each set of each exercise each week. As you will be mainly using free weights you could increase rep range up to as many as 30. Over time this will create muscular strength and endurance.

EXAMPLE 2
Working out using a time scale instead of using a rep count is another option. Start by training for 20 seconds on a set exercise. As your strength increases you may work out for as long as 60-90 seconds. This will also improve muscular strength and endurance.

TOP TIP
THINGS TO REMEMBER

- Start off slowly and as your strength increases, increase your speed.

- Maintain control and good posture throughout the exercise.

- Work hard on precision and not so much on speed.

- When exercising, never lock your limbs out totally.

FREE WEIGHTS ON THE SWISS BALL

1 LATERAL DOUBLE ARM RAISES

Muscles worked – Deltoids, shoulders.

THE START POSITION

Sit on the ball with a dumbbell in each hand by your hips. Keep your shoulders relaxed and your back straight. Without moving any other part of your body raise both arms level with your shoulders then lower the weights back down to your hips.

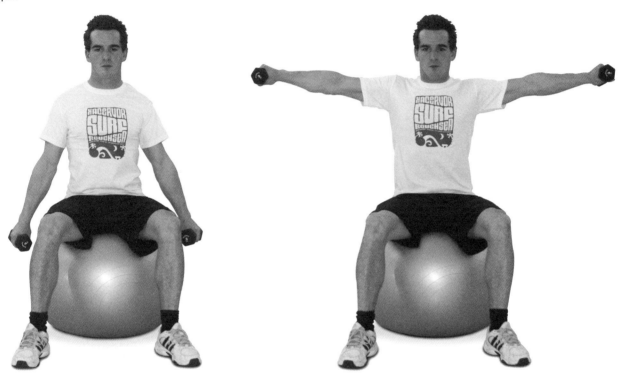

Keep your movements slow and controlled throughout the exercise and don't try too use too much weight too soon.

Repeat this for 6-8 reps initially

IMPROVES PADDLE POWER

2 CHEST PRESS ON THE BALL
Muscles worked – Pectorals, upper chest.

THE START POSITION
Lie flat on the ball with your hips raised and your back straight and parallel to the ground. With your feet hip width apart extend your arms towards the ceiling pressing the weights straight upwards. Keep the weights in line with your chest throughout the exercise and do not fully lock your arms at the top of the extension.

Bend your arms at the elbow lowering the weights to create a 90^0 angle then slowly press back up.

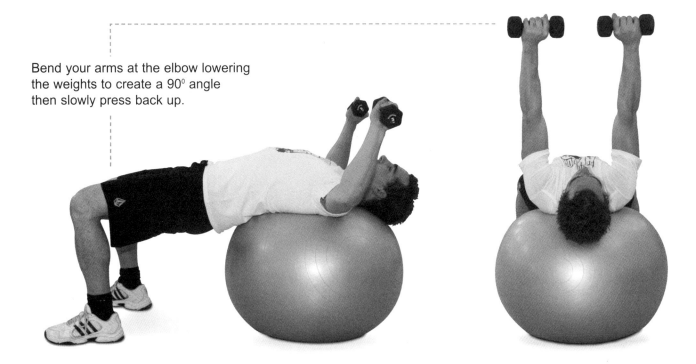

Keep your abdominals tight during the exercise and keep your movements slow and controlled throughout.

Repeat this for 6-8 reps initially.

IMPROVES PADDLE POWER

FREE WEIGHTS

3 SUPLINE PULLOVER PRESS
Muscles worked – Latissimus dorsi.

If you are new to the ball and weights use extra care with this exercise and use a very light weight until your balance has improved.

THE START POSITION
Lie flat on the ball with your hips raised and your feet hip width apart. Hold the weight tightly and raise it above your head. Keeping your arms slightly bent, lower the weight behind your head. Raise your arms back towards the ceiling in a slow controlled movement, returning to the start position .

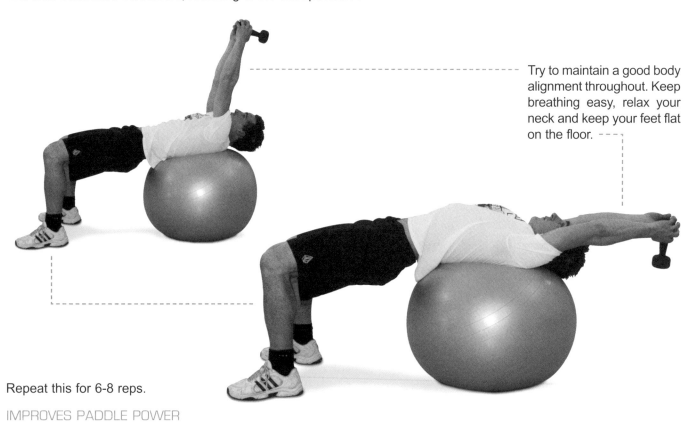

Try to maintain a good body alignment throughout. Keep breathing easy, relax your neck and keep your feet flat on the floor.

Repeat this for 6-8 reps.

IMPROVES PADDLE POWER

4 SHOULDER PRESS

Muscles worked – Deltoids.

THE START POSITION

Start by sitting on the ball holding the weights beside your shoulders ready to press upwards.

Push the weights up towards the ceiling with extra care not to lock your arms out. Slowly lower the weights back down to around ear level; your elbows should be in line with your shoulders.

Keep your back straight throughout the entire exercise and take care not to lock your arms completely

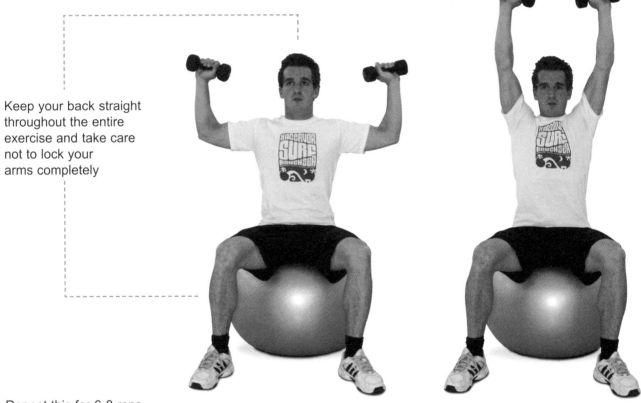

Repeat this for 6-8 reps.

IMPROVES PADDLE POWER

FREE WEIGHTS

5 REVERSE FLYE OVER THE BALL

Muscles worked – Trapezius and posterior deltoids.

THE START POSITION

Lie on top of the ball with your arms out in front of you and your back and shoulders relaxed. Raise your arms out sideways to shoulder level, with slightly bent elbows. Breath out and slowly lower the weights back to the start position.

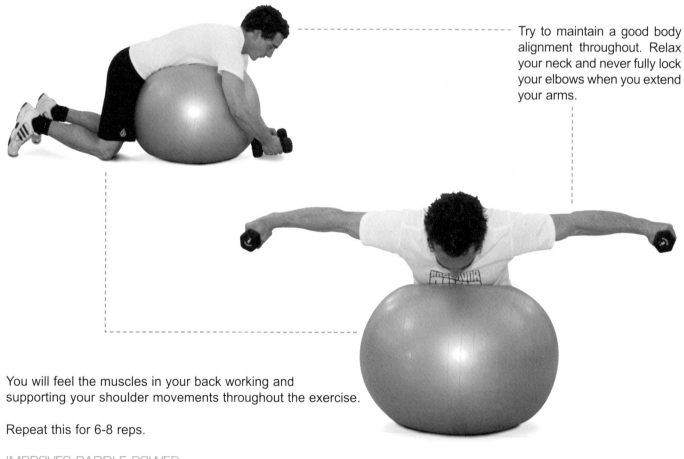

Try to maintain a good body alignment throughout. Relax your neck and never fully lock your elbows when you extend your arms.

You will feel the muscles in your back working and supporting your shoulder movements throughout the exercise.

Repeat this for 6-8 reps.

IMPROVES PADDLE POWER

6 TRICEP EXTENSIONS ON THE BALL
Muscles worked – Triceps

THE START POSITION
Start by putting your right knee on top of the ball, you can use your hand for a little extra support if you need it.

Hold the weight in your left hand. Your upper arm should be parallel to your back and your elbow should be bent creating a 90^0 angle. Keep your abdominals tight and your back straight.

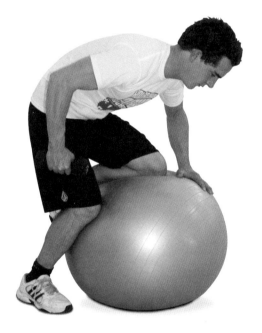 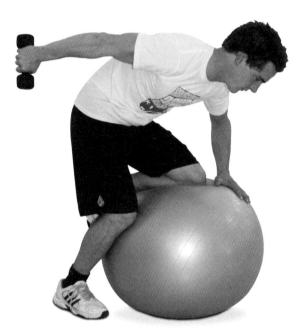

Straighten your arm in a smooth controlled motion to bring the weight level with your shoulder. Take care not to lock your arm out fully. You should feel the back of your arm contracting.

Repeat this for 6-8 reps on each side.

IMPROVES PADDLE POWER

FREE WEIGHTS

SWISS BALL

A BASIC WEIGHTS PROGRAMME

It's important to remember that as you start to increase the weights there will be an extra demand on your core strength. This in turn will put extra demands on your technique. It may be wise to increase your reps whilst using a low weight before moving on to slightly heavier weights.

PROGRAMME OF WEIGHTS FOR UPPER BODY STRENGTH

Outlined below is an example of a weights programme card that should be done at least twice a week. As the weeks progress add 2-3 reps to your workout. Try to avoid working out with weights 2 days in a row and try to space your training out for maximum recovery.

EXERCISE	WEIGHTS	REPS	WEIGHTS	REPS	WEIGHTS	REPS
LATERAL ARM RAISES						
CHEST PRESS						
LATERAL PULLOVER PRESS						
SHOULDER PRESS						
REVERSE FLYE						
TRICEP EXTENSION						
DATE						

AS WITH ANY TRAINING TAKE TIME TO COOL OFF AND STRETCH.
This will add flexibility to surfing and not stiffness

THIS PROGRAMME SHOULD BE COMBINED WITH A COMPREHENSIVE WORKOUT PROGRAMME FOR BEST RESULTS

ADDITIONAL BENEFITS OF RESISTANCE TRAINING

THE BENEFITS OF RESISTANCE TRAINING FOR SURFING

- IMPROVE MUSCLE SIZE AND STRENGTH
- IMPROVE THE STRENGTH OF LIGAMENTS AND TENDONS
- REDUCED BODY FAT
- IMPROVED POSTURE
- AID INJURY PREVENTION
- IMPROVED ALL OVER PADDLE POWER

Remember improving muscle strength takes time and a balanced all over body programme is vital for optimal strength and development. As a surfer muscle size is not that important. Surfing involves many dynamic movements and any weights training programme should mirror this. Speed agility and quickness are highly desirable skills for surfing. Increasing your muscle mass will not have a negative effect on your surfing providing you maintain a good flexibility and mobility programme.

CONSIDERATIONS FOR THE SURFER'S WEIGHT TRAINING PROGRAMME

1 IMPROVE UPPER BODY STRENGTH
Good all round improvements of a surfer's upper body strength can be highly beneficial for paddling out and pop-ups.

2 WEIGHT LOAD
Light to moderate weights will help you develop muscular strength and endurance (MSE) with additional gains in some muscle size (hypertrophy).

3 NUMBER OF REPS PER SET
For general improvements in MSE aim for a high number of reps per set. If you are new to resistance training 8-10 may be a good place to start, then over 6-8 weeks of regular training as many as 20 reps per set.

4 DON' T LIFT TOO FAST
Count 2-3 seconds on the way up and 3-4 seconds on the way down. This will ensure that you target the muscles you are aiming to work, therefore getting full benefit from the movement.

TOP TIP
THINGS TO REMEMBER

Remember, pumping iron day in day out can have a negative effect on your surfing movements. Stay flexible and supple!

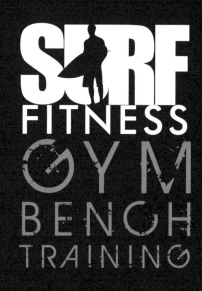

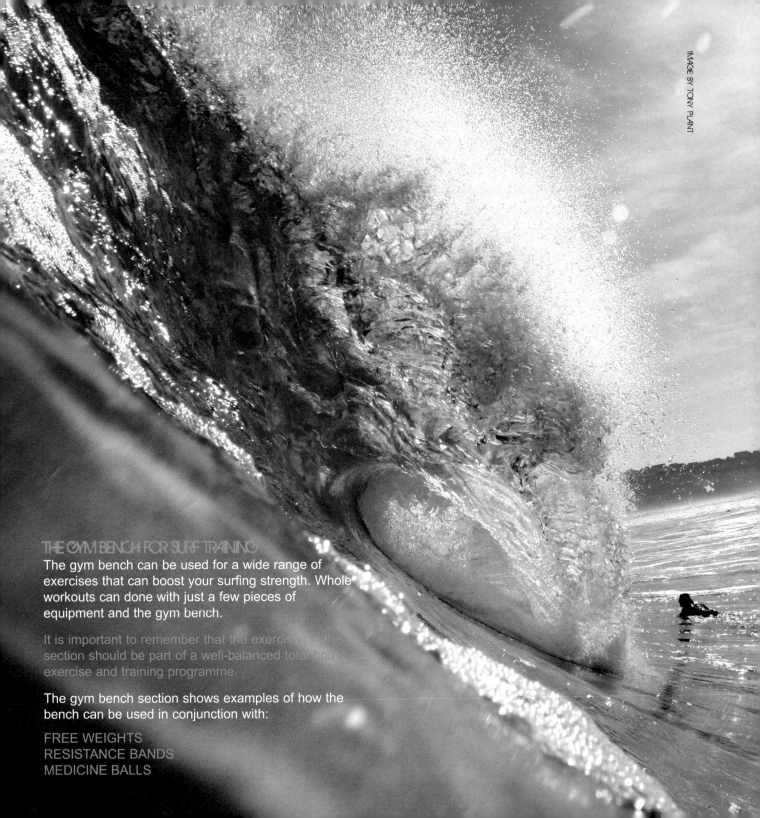

IMAGE BY TONY PLANT

THE GYM BENCH FOR SURF TRAINING

The gym bench can be used for a wide range of exercises that can boost your surfing strength. Whole workouts can done with just a few pieces of equipment and the gym bench.

It is important to remember that the exercises in this section should be part of a well-balanced total body exercise and training programme.

The gym bench section shows examples of how the bench can be used in conjunction with:

FREE WEIGHTS
RESISTANCE BANDS
MEDICINE BALLS

BENCH EXERCISES

1 TRICEP DIPS

Muscles worked – Triceps and deltoids.

Dips have been around for years. They are one of the simplest exercises yet one of the most effective for boosting your paddle power!

THE START POSITION

Start by placing feet hip width apart, bend your knees to about 90^0 and lower yourself down until your arms are bent to about 90^0. Pause briefly before slowly pushing back up until your arms are straight. Be careful not to lock the arms out fully when in the start position.

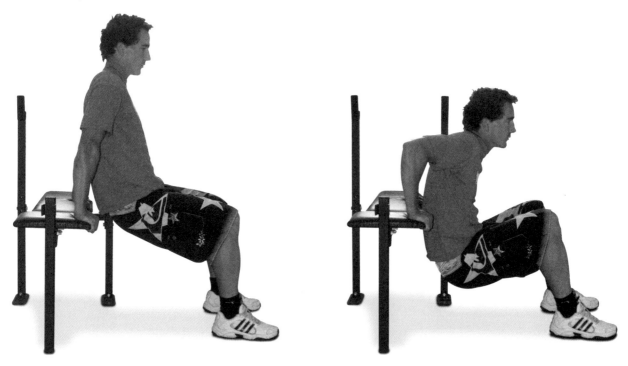

Repeat 6-8 reps, rest for 20 seconds then repeat. Throughout the exercise maintain a straight back and keep your head up.

IMPROVES PADDLE POWER

2 PLYOMETRIC PRESS UPS

Muscles worked – Pectorals, deltoids and triceps.

THE START POSITION

Start by placing both hands on the bench directly under your shoulders. Keeping your hands flat on the bench, slowly bend your arms to 90°. Using as much explosive power as possible push upwards and clap your hands together in mid air, landing with them back in the start position.

This is not a suitable exercise for a beginner. You should build up your strength doing normal press-ups first. You may also like to try a plyometric press-up on the floor before attempting the bench!

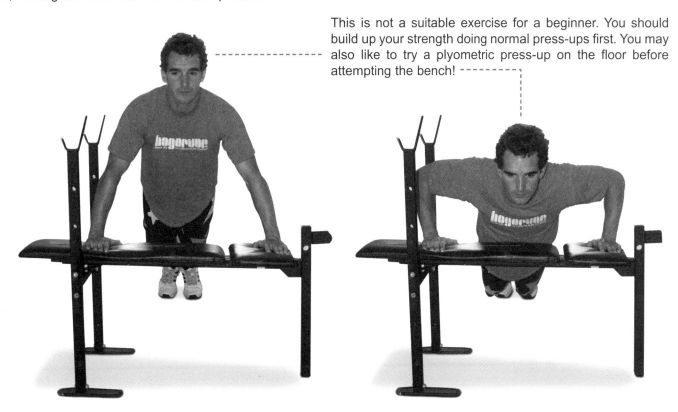

Press-ups are a great own body weight exercise for developing upper body strength and a strong core.

IMPROVES EXPLOSIVE POWER

3 REVERSE CRUNCH

Muscles worked – Lower rectus abdominus.

Great exercise for strengthening the lower abdominus which are used to stabilise the body during paddling.

THE START POSITION

Lie down on your back holding the top part of the bench to keep your body steady. Raise your feet in the air keeping your legs straight. Once your legs are in the air tighten your lower abdominals and push your hips upwards. Try to hold for 1-2 seconds before slowly lowering your legs back down. Keep your back flat on the bench throughout the exercise.

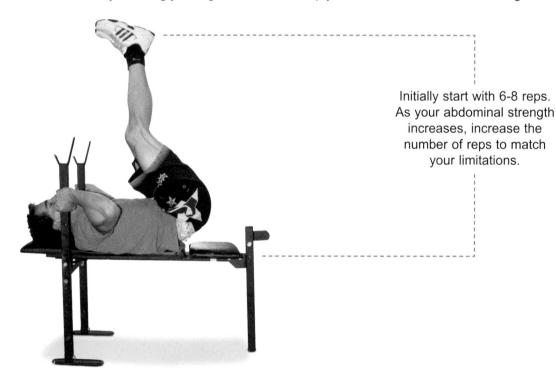

Initially start with 6-8 reps. As your abdominal strength increases, increase the number of reps to match your limitations.

You may wish to build up your strength with a basic reverse crunch on the floor.

IMPROVES CORE STRENGTH

1 FREE WEIGHTS – THE PEC FLYE

Muscles worked – pectorals.

THE START POSITION

Start by lying on your back on the bench with your feet on the floor. With your back flat on the bench, position the dumbbells directly above your chest. Slowly lower the weights out to the side until your hands are at shoulder level. Take care not to lock out your arms at the elbow, and keep your arms slightly bent.

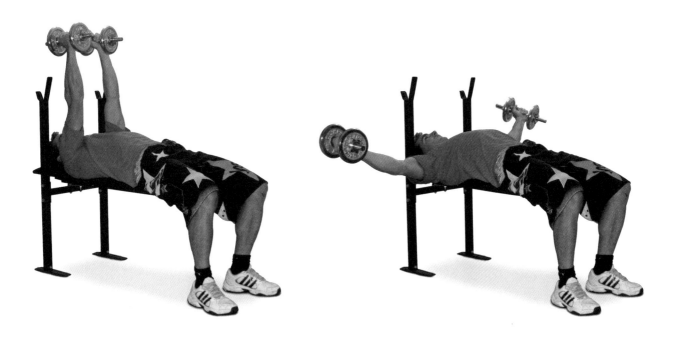

It is important to start with a super light weight with this one, as you get stronger you can increase the weight. A high-rep low weight is your best option to avoid injury.

Complete 8-12 reps to start then repeat.

KEEP YOUR MOVEMENTS FLUID AND CONTROLLED

2 SINGLE ARM UPRIGHT ROW

Muscles worked – Latissimus dorsi and rhomboids.

This is a great exercise for improving your paddle power. Try to use a medium-sized weight and maintain a good technique throughout the exercise. For more of a challenge try using the Swiss ball instead of the bench. This will challenge your core strength. Maintain focus on using your back muscles to pull the elbow through the movement with a slow and controlled technique.

THE START POSITION

Start by placing your left hand and knee on the bench, keeping your left foot on the floor. Hold a dumbbell in your right hand so it's hanging down towards the floor. Your back should be flat, straight and in line with the bench. Slowly pull the weight up towards your chest. Maintain a straight back and relaxed shoulders throughout the exercise.

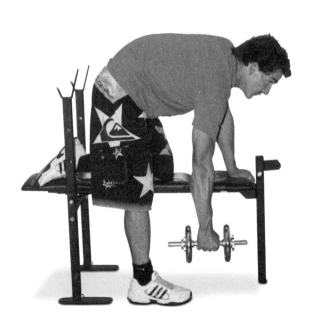 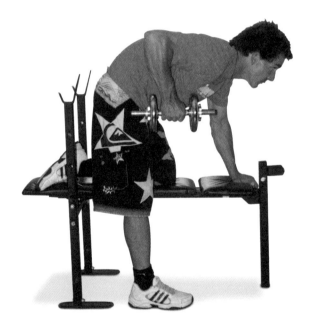

Repeat 8-12 reps to start, change sides and repeat.

TO SUPER SET THIS EXERCISE TRY 10 PRESS UPS AS SOON AS YOU HAVE FINISHED THE LAST REP!

3 TRICEP EXTENSION
Muscles worked – triceps.

The tricep muscle plays a major role in paddling. Keep your back straight during the movement; this will help you stay in the correct position.

THE START POSITION
Start by resting your left hand and knee on the bench. Hold the dumbbell in your right hand and leave your right foot on the floor. Slowly raise your right elbow bending your arm to about 90^0 so that your upper arm is parallel to the floor. Straighten your arm out behind you whilst flexing your tricep.

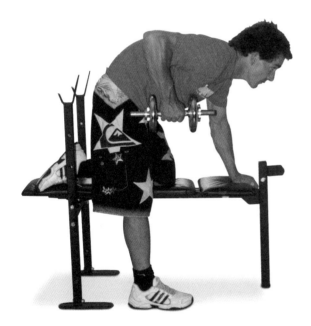 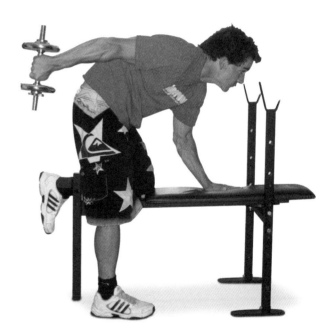

Repeat the movement 8-12 reps then repeat on the other arm.

TO CHALLENGE YOUR TRICEPS FURTHER TRY DOING A SET OF DIPS USING THE BENCH, SEE P116.

RESISTANCE BAND EXERCISES

1 LAND-BASED PADDLE WORKOUT – RESISTANCE BANDS
Using an extra long resistance band improves upper body strength.

THE START POSITION
Secure an extra long band to the bench and stand well back, stretching the band fully to generate full resistance. Lean forwards and paddle in a movement that resembles front crawl.

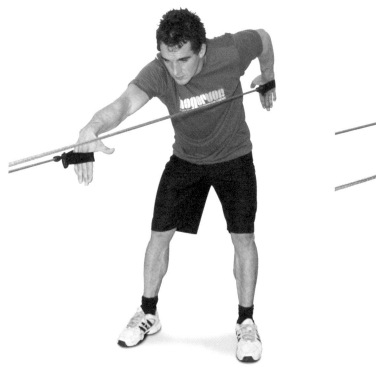
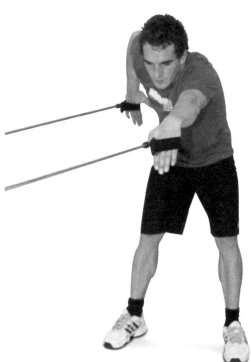

Although a 10 minute paddle at an average pace 2-3 times a week will be of use, you may also wish to break the workout down into sections in the same way you would in the pool.

IMPROVES PADDLE POWER AND STAMINA

2 UPRIGHT ROW

Using a smaller resistance band. Muscles worked – Deltoids and triceps.

This is a good exercise for the shoulder muscles and will increase your paddling power and strength.

Make sure that the bench you secure the resistance band to is heavy enough not to lift up during the exercise.

THE START POSITION

Start by fixing your band low down near the floor. Stand with feet hip width apart and your legs slightly bent. Keep your back straight throughout the exercise

Hold the bands by the handles, resting them on your thighs. Slowly raise hands upwards to chest level. Lead with your elbows pointing them upwards.

Slowly lower your hands and return to the starting position.

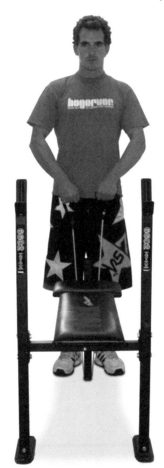
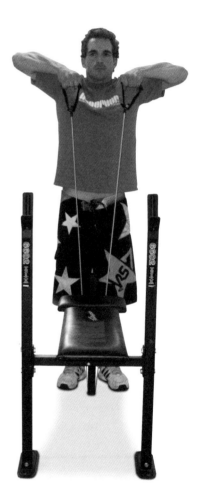

Try working for 60 seconds then repeat after 30 seconds rest.

IMPROVES PADDLE POWER

3 FRONT SHOULDER RAISE

Using a smaller resistance band. Muscles worked – Deltoids.

The deltoid (shoulder muscle) can be broken into three sections or parts: the posterior (back of shoulder), the anterior (front of shoulder) and the medial and lateral (middle or top section).

A well-balanced exercise programme should work all of these areas. This can help you maintain over all shoulder strength and help to boost your paddle endurance.

THE START POSITION

Start by attaching the band to the bottom area of the bench. Position yourself with your feet hip width apart, holding the band handles by your hips.

Straddle the bench and slowly raise the band up to shoulder level.

Hold for 1-2 seconds then slowly return to start the position and repeat the exercise.

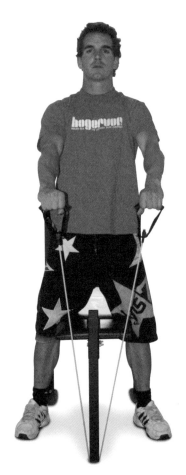
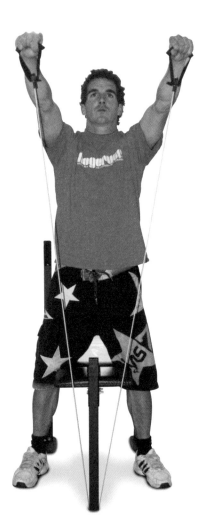

Try working for 60 seconds then repeat after 30 seconds rest.

IMPROVES PADDLE POWER

1 MEDICINE BALL EXERCISES – SUPINE PULLOVER PRESS

Muscles worked – Latissimus dorsi (sides of back). This area of the back plays a major role in swimming and surf paddling.

THE START POSITION

Lie flat on the bench with your feet on the floor either side of the bench. Raise the medicine ball upwards from your chest with both hands and lower it back behind your head, stopping when it's about level with your ears.

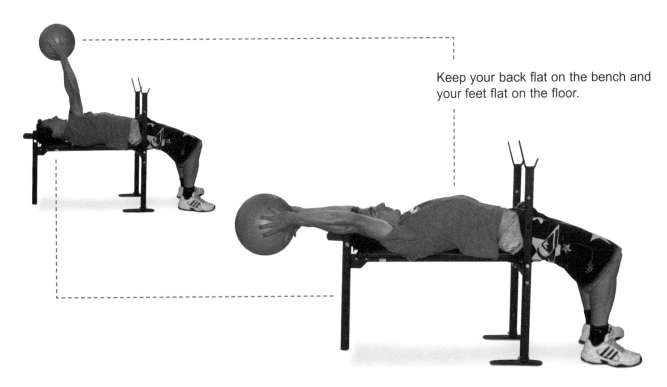

Keep your back flat on the bench and your feet flat on the floor.

Hold for 1-2 seconds and return to the start position, repeat 8-12 times. This exercise can be done on the Swiss ball for additional gains in core strength.

IMPROVES PADDLE POWER AND STAMINA

BENCH EXERCISES

2 SEATED TRICEPS EXTENSION
Muscles worked – Triceps.

THE START POSITION
Start by sitting on the end of the bench with your feet flat on the floor. Hold the ball with both hands, extend your arms out and raise the ball above your head so your wrists, elbows and shoulders are vertically aligned with each other. Slowly lower the ball behind your head keeping your elbows stationary.

Slowly extend your arms returning the ball to the vertical position.

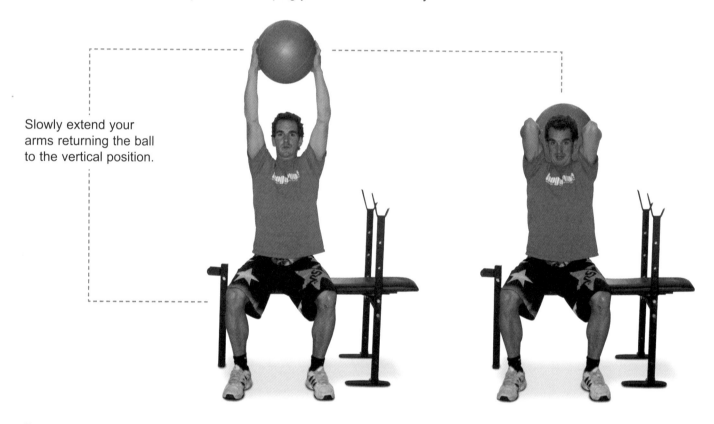

Repeat 8-12 times taking care not to use too heavy a medicine ball too quickly.

IMPROVES PADDLE POWER AND STAMINA

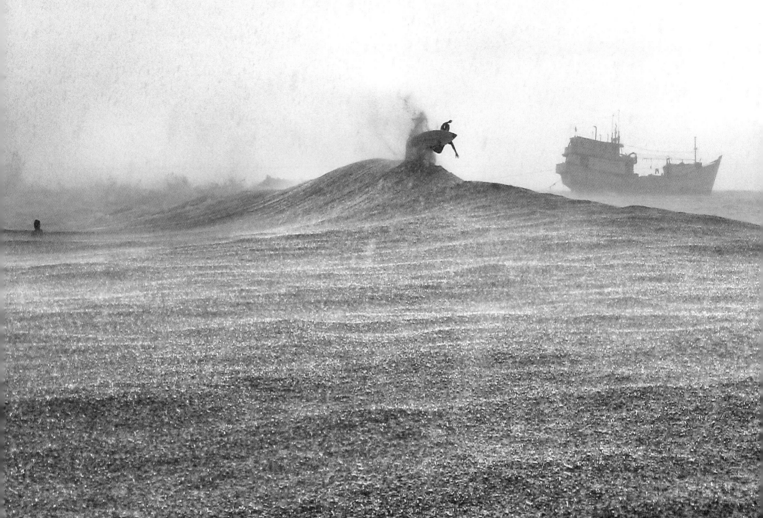

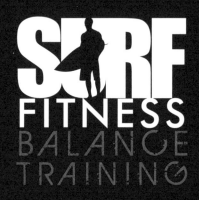

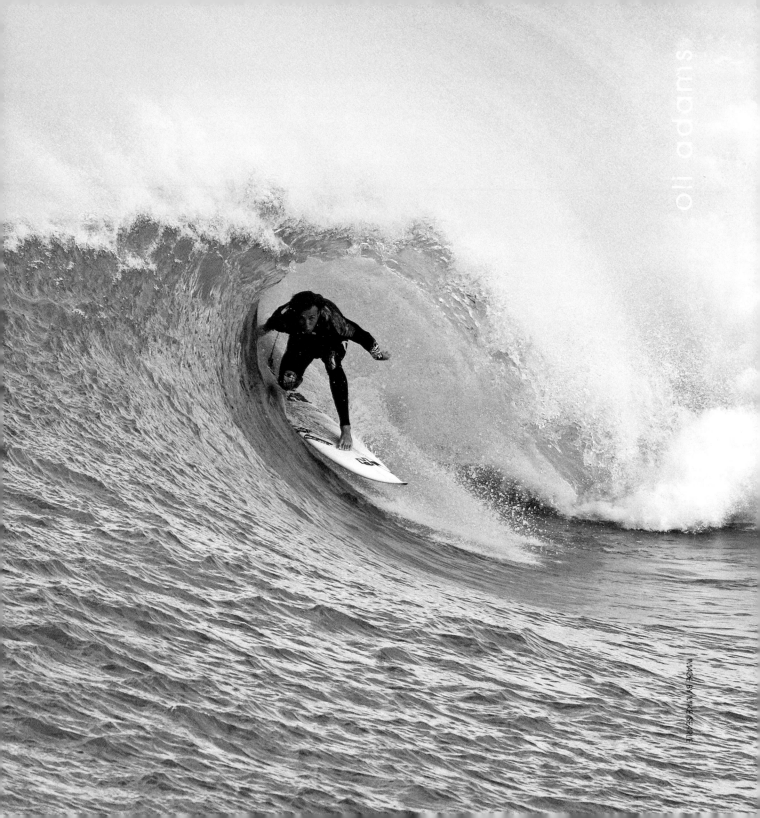

BALANCE
TRAINING

PROPRIOCEPTIVE TRAINING AND TIPS FOR SURFERS

Proprioceptive training can improve a surfer's strength, coordination, muscular balance and muscle reaction times, allowing you to surf with more confidence and flair.

This form of training can also aid injury prevention during sporting activity.

For you as a surfer to fully understand the key elements of balance training it's important to take into account that as the body carries out athletic movements, your overall muscular activity and the range of movement at your joints are all the products of sensory nerve activity. This activity is received, and then acted on by your brain and spinal cord, otherwise known as the central nervous system. The central nervous system gets the information it needs from three other subsystems within your body – your somatosensory system your vestibular system and your visual system.

THE SOMATOSENSORY SYSTEM'S MAIN ROLE

The somatosensory system contains nerves located in the skin, muscle and tendon junctions and joints. It can detect touch, pressure, joint motion and position. By engaging in balance training, the somatosensory system can be improved, thus improving surfer's joint movement and body movements.

In addition to the somatosensory system, the vestibular system, which is used to pick up information using vestibules and semicircular canals of the inner ear, helps to maintain overall body posture and balance. This works together with the visual system and plays a major role in the maintenance of balance. You can gain a full appreciation of this by simply standing on one leg!

If you are unable to surf as often as you like, balance training can be of utmost importance in maintaining your surfing ability.

IMPORTANT TO REMEMBER

Any balance equipment is unstable by nature. Take extra care when starting out – when using the equipment keep your back straight, contract your abdominals and use your core strength to stabilise your movements.

BALANCE TRAINING KIT

INDO BOARD

The Indo board is a great bit of kit, and has a variety of uses for surfing strength and conditioning. You can use the Indo board on its own or with other training equipment.

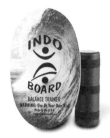

BALANCE/INFLATABLE DISC

These are great for balance training and strengthening your legs, knees, ligaments and joints.

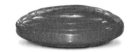

THE BOSU

My fav! The BOSU can be used both sides up for strength , core and balance training.

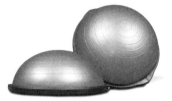

WOBBLE BOARDS

These come in different shapes and sizes. They can aid balance and are great for ankle strength and improving knee strength.

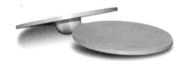

THE SWISS BALL

There are some restrictions with the ball and most balance training can only be done at advanced level.

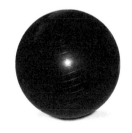

BALANCE TRAINING WITH THE SWISS BALL

Although there are limitations to balance training using the Swiss ball,
there is room for the Swiss ball in any surfer's balance training programme.
Not all exercises may be suitable for beginners but with practice
your proprioceptive balance skills will soon improve.

1 KNEELING BALANCE ON THE SWISS BALL
Difficulty Level – Beginner

THE START POSITION
Start by kneeling on the ball with your knees slightly apart. Keep your back straight and your head up. Use your arms to balance yourself and avoid the temptation to sit back on the ball. Until you feel comfortable balancing on the ball you may wish to use a training partner to support you.

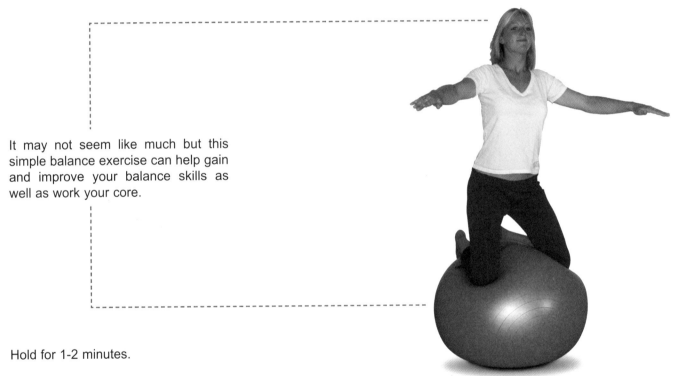

It may not seem like much but this simple balance exercise can help gain and improve your balance skills as well as work your core.

Hold for 1-2 minutes.

IMPROVES BALANCE AND CORE STRENGTH

ADVANCING THE EXERCISE
Once you feel comfortable kneeling on the ball then you can move on to light weights training.

BALANCE TRAINING

2 LATERAL RAISES KNEELING ON THE SWISS BALL
Difficulty Level – Intermediate

THE START POSITION
Start by kneeling on the Swiss ball with a dumbbell in each hand. Don't try to be a hero, start with a small weight and build up to a heavier weight.

Once you are steady try some lateral raises. Start the exercise movement with the weights by your hips. Keeping your back straight and your head up slowly lift the weights to shoulder level then repeat.

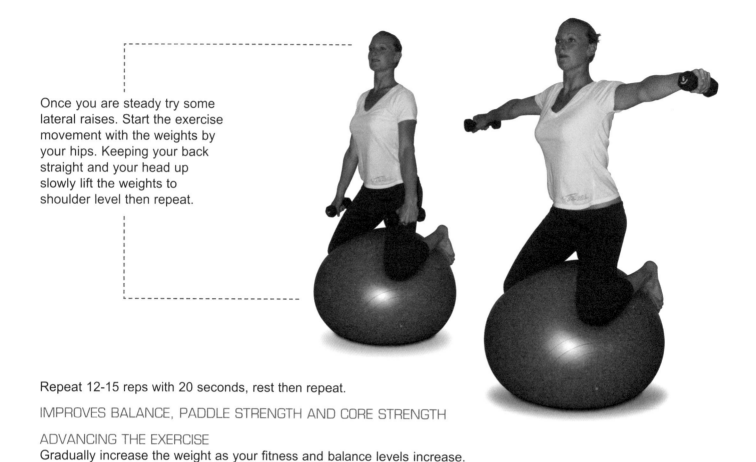

Repeat 12-15 reps with 20 seconds, rest then repeat.

IMPROVES BALANCE, PADDLE STRENGTH AND CORE STRENGTH

ADVANCING THE EXERCISE
Gradually increase the weight as your fitness and balance levels increase.

3 BICEPS CURL TO SHOULDER PRESS KNEELING ON THE SWISS BALL
Difficulty Level – Advanced

THE START POSITION
Start by kneeling on the Swiss ball holding a dumbbell in each hand (you may need the help of a training partner to start the exercise correctly). In one fluid motion, lift the dumbbells to shoulder height bending your arm at the elbow and then fully extend your arms pressing the weights above your head.

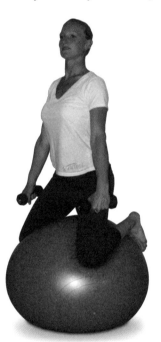 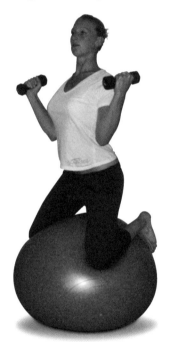 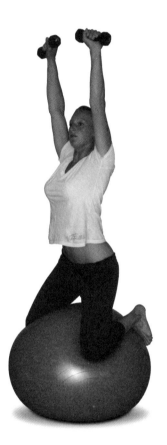

Repeat 10-15 reps with 20 seconds, rest then repeat.

IMPROVES BALANCE, PADDLE STRENGTH AND CORE STRENGTH

EXTRA SAFETY NOTE
Make sure that you have plenty of space and a safe training area. Take care not to lock your arms out fully when extended.

BALANCE TRAINING

4 MEDICINE BALL THROWS KNEELING ON THE SWISS BALL
Difficulty Level – Advanced

THE START POSITION
Start by kneeling on the Swiss ball facing your training partner. Initially you may want to use a light ball e.g. a tennis ball or a football, then progress to a lightweight medicine ball.

This exercise involves passing the ball to and fro while kneeling on the Swiss ball.

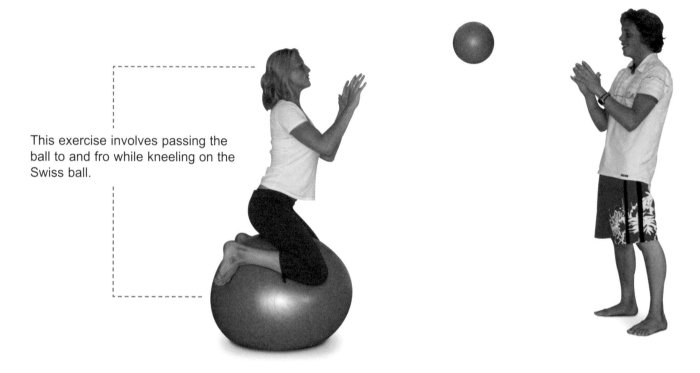

Repeat 10 reps with 20 seconds, rest then repeat.

IMPROVES BALANCE, PADDLE STRENGTH AND CORE STRENGTH

ADVANCING THE EXERCISE
Gradually increase the weight of the ball and the distance passed as your fitness and balance levels increase.

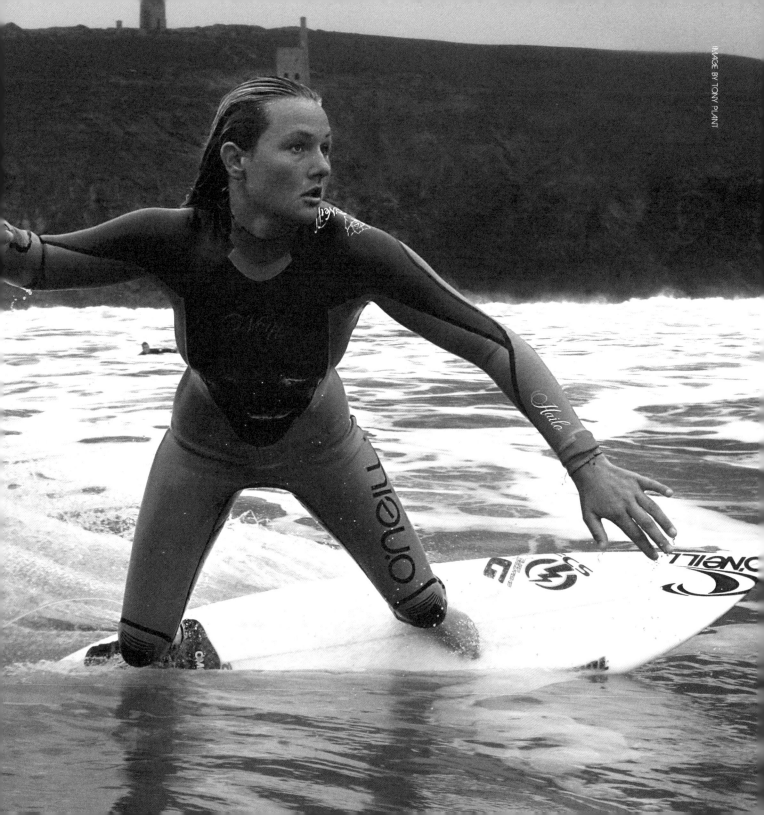

BALANCE TRAINING WITH THE WOBBLE BOARD

Wobble boards have been around for some time. They were used in some of the very first studies looking at the potential for balance improvement in sporting and athletic movements.

Simple balance training exercises can be carried out using the wobble board for additional surfing strength. Most wobble boards are relatively inexpensive and are sold everywhere. By using wobble boards a surfer can increase ankle and knee strength over time, and thus aid injury prevention.

They are extremely versatile and can be used in conjunction with other kit like the Swiss ball. It's a great way to improve core strength and can fit in to a surfer's well-balanced weekly training programme.

Before attempting this exercise find a non-slippery surface for your board to rest on. If you have never used a wobble board before then it may well take some time before you are ready to start basic movements on the board.

1 WOBBLE BOARD SQUATS
Difficulty Level - Basic

THE START POSITION
Start by standing on the wobble board feet about hip width apart and your shoulders back. Slowly shift hips backwards and descend. Lower your upper body until the legs are at a 90^0 angle then slowly return to starting position.

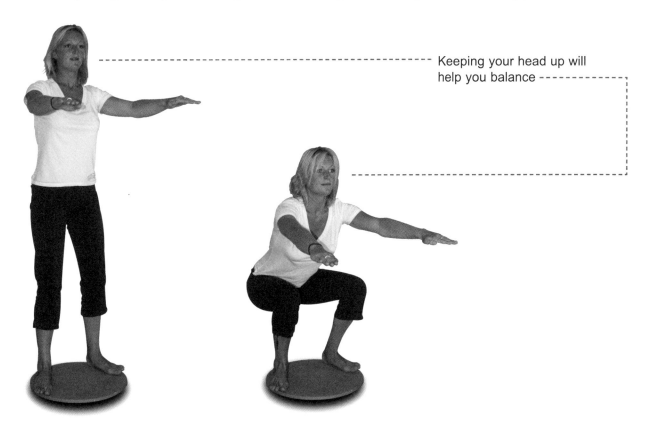

Keeping your head up will help you balance

Repeat 10-15 reps with 20 seconds rest then repeat.

IMPROVES QUADRICEPS, HAMSTRINGS AND JOINT STRENGTH

2 ADVANCED WOBBLE BOARD SQUATS USING WEIGHTS
Difficulty Level – Advanced

THE START POSITION
Start by standing on the board with your arms down and the dumbbells or medicine ball at about hip height. Lower yourself to a 90^0 squat and extend both arms out in front of you, keeping them straight.

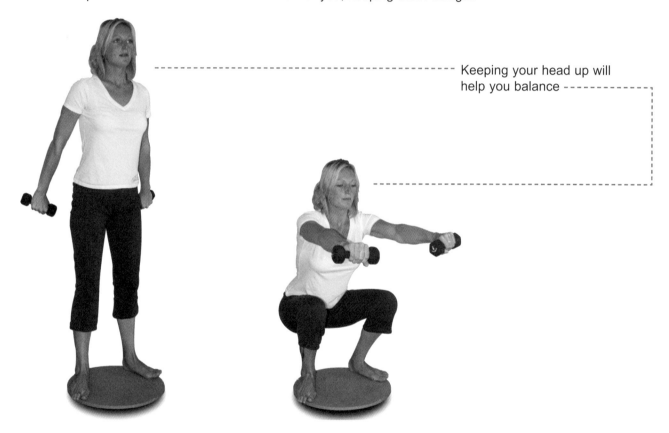

Keeping your head up will help you balance

Repeat 10 reps with 20 seconds rest then repeat.

IMPROVES QUADRICEPS, HAMSTRINGS AND JOINT STRENGTH

3 BALANCE TRAINING WITH THE WOBBLE BOARD
Difficulty Level – Advanced

THE START POSITION
Start by standing on the edge of the board, close your eyes and squat slightly. By closing your eyes you will challenge your somatosensory system skills further.

It is advisable not to attempt advanced exercises if you are a beginner on the wobble board.

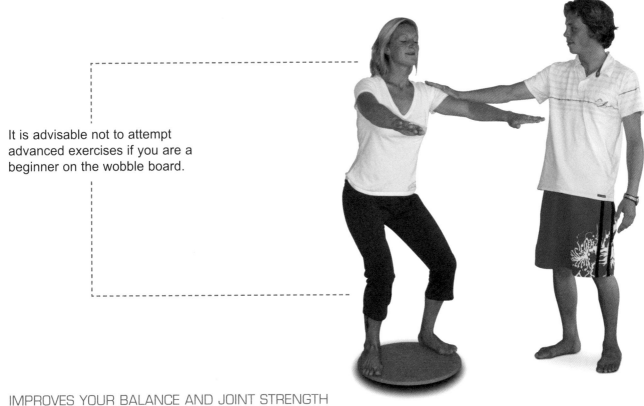

IMPROVES YOUR BALANCE AND JOINT STRENGTH

ADVANCING THE EXERCISE
Try getting your training partner to lightly push you whilst you balance with your eyes closed. For this to be effective they should alternate where they push you. You could also try using weights or a medicine ball.

BALANCE TRAINING WITH THE INFLATABLE DISC

The inflatable disc can be used in a similar way to the wobble board but due to its construction and size it's slightly more versatile. Exercises using the inflatable disc alone can be extremely beneficial for strengthening a surfer's knees, hips and ankles as well as improving general overall leg strength. It can also be used in conjunction with other apparatus like the Indo board and Swiss ball and as it is relatively inexpensive and portable it's a great bit of kit.

During many surfing movements the knee acts as a shock absorber along with the spine. The knee is a highly complex joint, and the bones are all linked by ligaments, also known as a freely moveable joint or synovial joints these joints can often be at high risk from injury. The disc lunge is a very good exercise for ligament strength. This will help maintain strength through a surfing movement from beginners' moves or advanced like the roundhouse cutback on a short-board. A basic turn on a longboard will also demand knee strength and the more you are able to drop knee, the more the knee can be put under strain.

As mentioned previously, the somatosensory system is aided by two other systems, the vestibular system and the visual system. The vestibular system, which picks up information from the vestibules and semicircular canals of the inner ear, maintains overall posture and balance. The visual system also plays a large role in the maintenance of balance, so to improve balance further try lunging on the disc with your eyes closed!

BEFORE STARTING

If you are new to exercise, the following exercises can be done initially without the inflatable balance disc in order for you to build up your joint strength.

The inflatable balance disc can easily cause injury if it is not used correctly. You will inevitably wobble at first, and it is important that your posture is correct to avoid injury.

1 THE BASIC LUNGE ON THE INFLATABLE DISC
Difficulty Level – Intermediate

THE START POSITION
Start the exercise with your feet a stride's width apart and one foot on the disc. Slowly lower the knee of your back leg until both are at a 90⁰ angle, then slowly push back up to the start position. Take extra care not to hyper-extend the knee of your front leg over or past your toes. Maintain a smooth and controlled movement throughout the exercise.

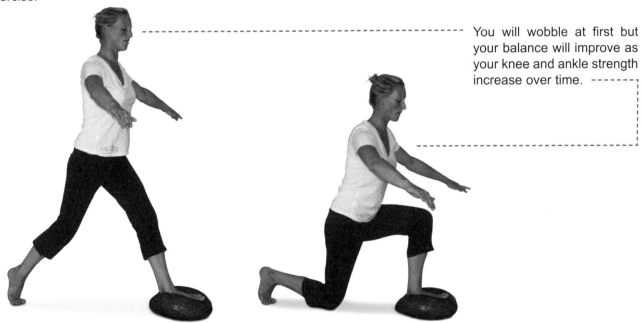

You will wobble at first but your balance will improve as your knee and ankle strength increase over time.

Repeat 5 reps on one leg, then change and repeat on the opposite leg.

IMPROVES QUADRICEPS, HAMSTRINGS AND BASIC BALANCE

ADVANCING THE EXERCISE
Once you feel comfortable lunging on the inflatable balance disc, you could try using weights whilst lunging. See the next exercise.

2 THE BASIC LUNGE ON THE INFLATABLE DISC WITH PRESS
Difficulty Level – Intermediate

THE START POSITION
Start the exercise with your feet a stride's width apart, one foot on the disc and the dumbbells at shoulder height. Slowly bend your legs until they are both at a 90° angle. At the same time press the dumbbells straight up above your head. Once you have reached a 90° angle push back up and lower the dumbbells to the start position. Take extra care not to hyper-extend the knee of your front leg over or past your toes. Maintain a smooth and controlled movement throughout the exercise.

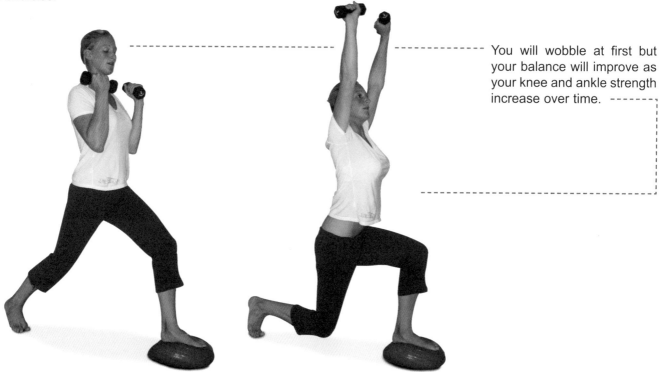

You will wobble at first but your balance will improve as your knee and ankle strength increase over time.

Repeat 5 reps on one leg, then change and repeat on the opposite leg.

IMPROVES QUADRICEPS, SHOULDER STRENGTH, HAMSTRINGS AND BASIC BALANCE

3 LATERAL RAISES AND SEATED LEG LIFTS WITH THE SWISS BALL
Difficulty Level – Intermediate

THE START POSITION
Start by sitting on the Swiss ball with your back straight and shoulders relaxed, and light weights in both hands. Place one foot on your inflatable balance disc. Once you feel comfortable extend your other leg horizontally. At the same time raise weights laterally to shoulder level.

Try to keep your foot centralised on the inflatable balance disc throughout the exercise. Complete 5 leg lifts on one side then repeat on the other side.

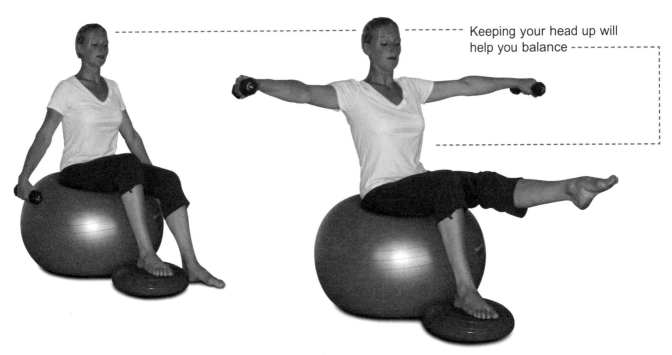

Keeping your head up will help you balance

CHALLENGES CORE STRENGTH AND BALANCE SKILLS

ADVANCING THE EXERCISE
Once you feel comfortable with the lateral raises try adding front raises and shoulder presses to your set.

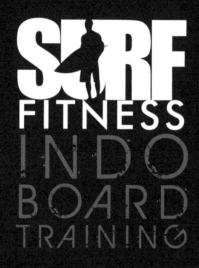

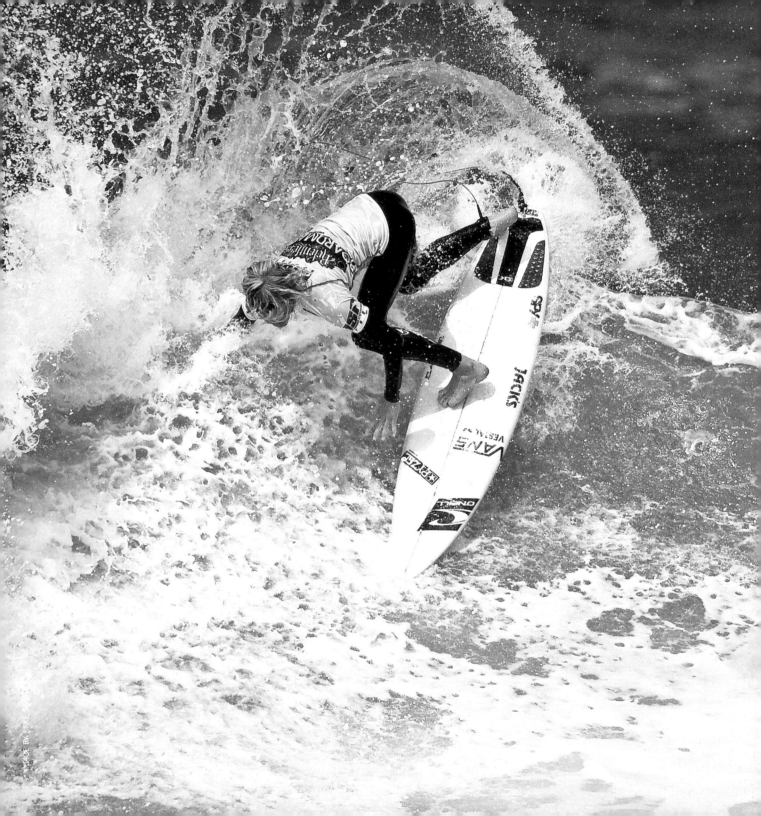

INDO BOARD

TRAINING

BALANCE TRAINING USING THE INDO BOARD

THE INDO BOARD - MULTI JOINT TRAINING AND BALANCE

In most sports athletes are required to use a variety of complex movements, and surfing is no different. Training should be performed in a sport specific manner if possible and that's where the benefits of Indo board training come in.

To maximize training time and function, multi joint exercises such as squats and lunges are usually more efficient than single joint exercises as they do not isolate a single joint activity. Because multi-joint exercises on the Indo are mostly performed in a slow, controlled motion the likelihood of injury is greatly reduced.

Single joint action is uncommon in surfing movements but does

occur. Single joint balance training, as the name suggests, focuses on the muscle groups surrounding one joint. They are beneficial to the surfer but can be very time consuming.

Many sports depend exclusively on an athlete's control of centre of gravity and the ability to balance during the sport's activity. As soon as the athlete loses balance movement is then lost! Surfing is one of these sports!

The Indo board has to be one of the most popular balance training packs available to the surfer to date and when used with the IndoFLO2 cushion it has to be one of the most versatile.

To fully appreciate the benefits of the Indo board you will need to put in a certain amount of practice, but after a short time you should be

ready for even basic movements that can boost your surfing fitness.

INDO BOARD WITH FREE WEIGHTS

There is a vast range of exercises that can be done on the Indo board using free weights that will aid and boost your paddle and surfing strength.

Working out while standing on the Indo will challenge your core strength while also making the movements much more challenging. Be sure to maintain the correct technique throughout all movements.

ADVANCED GAINS

Advanced gains in muscular balance and muscular fitness require flexibility, strength, muscular endurance, power and speed. The Indo board should be used as part of a well-rounded training programme involving all of these components. The regular use of an Indo board will help in overall athleticism and coordination, prevent injuries and best of all enhance and improve your surfing performance whilst having fun at the same time.

TOP TIP
THINGS TO REMEMBER

Any balance equipment is unstable by nature. Take extra care when starting out, use a partner initially if needed to help you balance. When using the equipment keep your back straight, contract your abdominals and use your core strength to stabilise your movements.

INDO BOARD EXERCISES

1 BASIC INDO SQUAT
Difficulty Level – Beginner

Regular Indo squats will allow you to develop an improved stance on the Indo board which will translate directly into your surfing. As with the wobble board, the Indo board will help generate strength in the ankles, knees and major muscles of the legs.

Before your first squat be sure that you have developed a good base of balance on the Indo board to work from. Once you have this then you are ready to start.

THE START POSITION
Start the exercise balancing on the Indo board with your feet hip width apart. Looking forward and keeping your head up throughout the exercise will help you balance.

Once you feel ready, slowly bend your knees and lower yourself into a squat, extending your arms out in front of you to aid your balance.

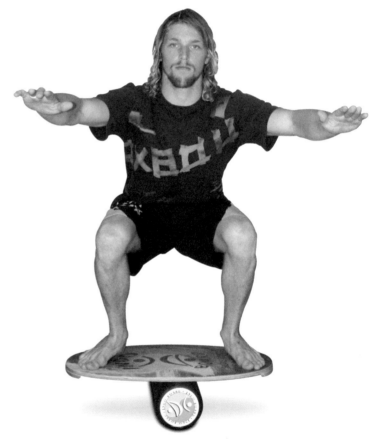

Repeat this as many times as you can before fatigue sets in, then rest and repeat.

IMPROVES QUADRICEPS, HAMSTRINGS AND JOINT STRENGTH

ADVANCING THE EXERCISE
You can advance this exercise further by using a medicine ball – see the next exercise in this section.

2 INDO SQUAT WITH MEDICINE BALL
Difficulty Level – Beginner

As with the basic Indo squat, before your first squat be sure that you have developed a good base of balance on the Indo board to work from.

THE START POSITION
Start the exercise balancing on the Indo board with your feet hip width apart. Hold the medicine ball in front of you at waist height with both hands. Slowly bend your knees and lower yourself into a squat. Keeping your arms straight and your head up, extend your arms out in front of you raising the medicine ball to around shoulder height.

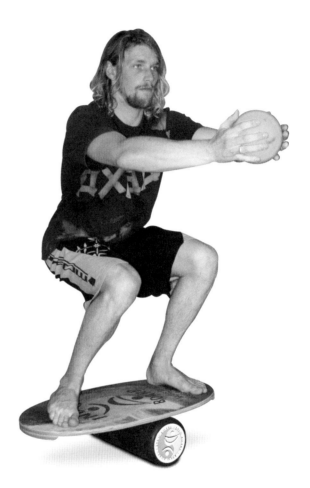

Repeat this as many times as you can before fatigue sets in, then rest and repeat.

IMPROVES QUADRICEPS, HAMSTRINGS, CORE, PADDLE AND JOINT STRENGTH

ADVANCING THE EXERCISE
You can advance this exercise further by using weights instead of the medicine ball, gradually increasing the weight as your fitness increases.

3 BASIC LATERAL RAISE
Difficulty Level – Beginner to Intermediate

THE START POSITION
Start with feet hip width apart, a good upright body position and the weights by your hips. Slowly raise the weights upwards keeping them in line with the body to around shoulder level.

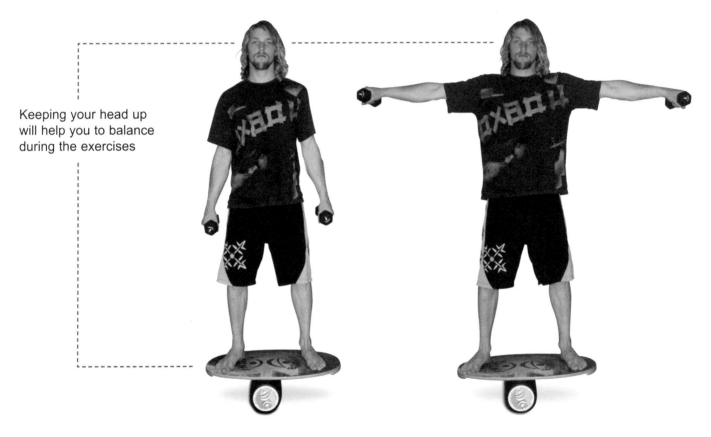

Keeping your head up will help you to balance during the exercises

Repeat 8-12 reps with 20 seconds rest then repeat.

IMPROVES BALANCE, PADDLE STRENGTH AND CORE STRENGTH

4 BICEP CURL INTO A SHOULDER PRESS
Difficulty Level – Beginner to Intermediate

THE START POSITION
Start with your feet hip width apart and the weights by your hips. Bending your arms at your elbows, slowly raise the weights towards your shoulders with your palms facing inwards. Twist the weights so your palms are facing outwards and shoulder press them upwards.

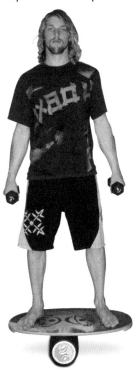 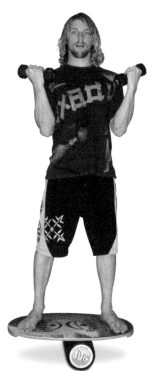 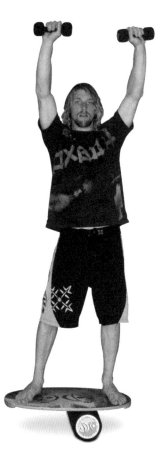

Be sure not to lock your arms straight at the end of the movement. Slowly reverse the exercise to bring the weights back to the start position.

Repeat 8-12 reps with 20 seconds rest then repeat.

IMPROVES BALANCE, PADDLE STRENGTH AND CORE STRENGTH

INDO BOARD EXERCISES

5 INDO BOARD PRESS UPS
Difficulty Level – Intermediate

Indo board press-ups will challenge your core further and at the same time boost your lower back strength.

THE START POSITION
Start the exercise as you would a normal press-up only this time place your hands at either end of the Indo board. Keep your back straight and feet slightly apart. Slowly lower into a press-up movement and just before your chest reaches the Indo board push back up.

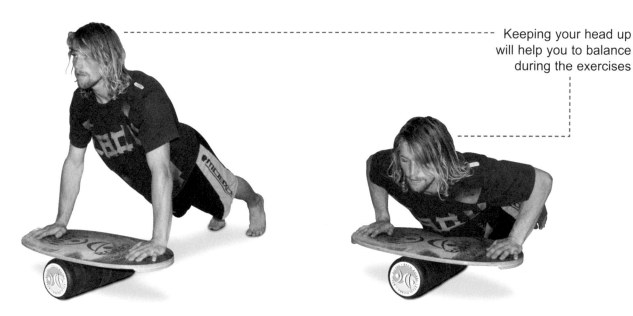

Keeping your head up will help you to balance during the exercises

Repeat 8-12 reps with 20 seconds rest then repeat as many times as possible.

IMPROVES BALANCE, PADDLE STRENGTH AND CORE STRENGTH

ADVANCING THE EXERCISE
You can advance this exercise further by raising your feet off the ground when executing the press-up. For an example see the next exercise.

6 INDO BOARD PRESS-UPS WITH THE SWISS BALL
Difficulty Level – Advanced

As your fitness levels and balance improve this exercise is a good way of advancing the Indo board press-up.

THE START POSITION
Start the exercise by placing both hands on the Indo board as before and place both feet together on the Swiss ball. Once you are stable begin the exercise. Keep your back straight and your feet together. Slowly lower into a press-up movement and just before your chest reaches the Indo board push back up.

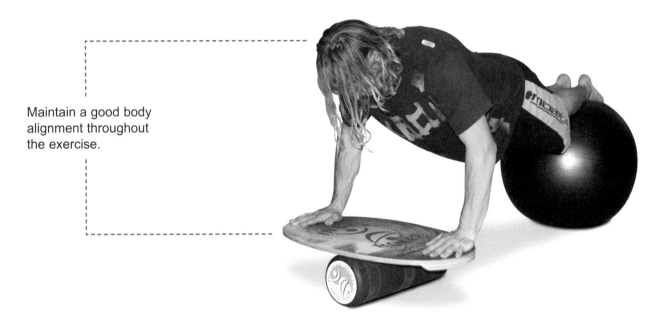

Maintain a good body alignment throughout the exercise.

REMEMBER THIS IS AN ADVANCED EXERCISE AND SHOULD ONLY BE CARRIED OUT ONCE YOU HAVE REACHED A GOOD LEVEL OF CORE AND UPPER BODY STRENGTH.

Repeat 8-12 reps with 20 seconds rest then repeat as many times as possible.

IMPROVES BALANCE, PADDLE STRENGTH AND CORE STRENGTH

TRANSFER BALANCE EXERCISE

Transfer balance exercises can add a new dimension to your training session. The advantage of introducing a second person into the exercise is that it adds a level of anticipation you cannot get working out on your own. Having to move instinctively to counter your partner's movements will help increase your reaction speed alongside your fitness.

BASIC BALANCE TRANSFER EXERCISE
Difficulty Level – Intermediate to Advanced

THE START POSITION
Start with your feet hip width apart on the Indo board about 2-3 metres away from your partner. Throw the medicine ball to your partner whilst maintaining your balance.

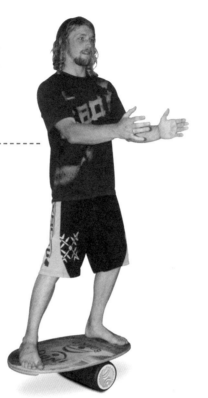
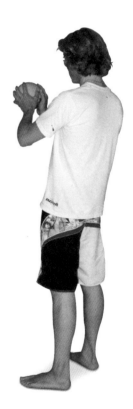

Try to use a wide range of movements from left to right whilst on the Indo board. This will improve your ability to transfer balance from one side to the other.

Repeat 8-12 reps with 20 seconds rest then repeat as many times as possible.

IMPROVES BALANCE, CORE STRENGTH AND REACTION SPEED

ADVANCING THE EXERCISE
You can advance this exercise further by squatting on the Indo board as you throw the medicine ball.

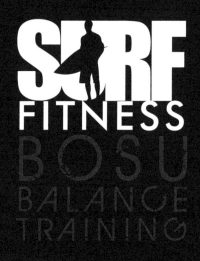

THE
BOSU BALL
FOR SURFING STRENGTH

As a surfer wishing to gain additional surfing strength the BOSU can be a great training tool. The BOSU can be used for a whole range of training types that can aid surfing performance and strength. Like the Indo Board the BOSU is a great training tool for any surfer wishing to improve dynamic balance, agility and core stabilisation.

For more info on the BOSU balance trainer go to www.bosu.com. If you're new to the BOSU there is an owner's manual guiding you through basic movements to advanced exercises.

ben skindog skinner

BOSU BALANCE TRAINING

1 PUSH-UP WITH PLATFORM TILT

The goal of this exercise is to challenge your upper body strength and core stabilisation. If you are looking for any improvement in your paddle strength, this is a great exercise when combined with a total body training programme.

THE START POSITION
Turn the BOSU dome side down so that the platform is facing up. Begin in either a press-up position, or a kneeling press-up position (depending on your level of fitness), with your hands grasping the recessed grips on the sides of the platform. With straight arms, align your chest over the centre of the platform. Bend your elbows, lowering your chest towards your hands and press back up into the start position. Make sure you maintain a good body alignment.

Keeping your elbows extended, tilt the platform slightly to one side allowing your entire body to tilt. Keep your core muscles contracted for stabilisation. Tilt the platform back to a level position.

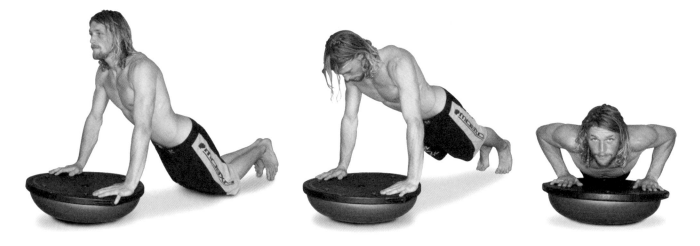

Alternate a single push-up with a tilt to one side. Repeat the push-up and tilt to the other side. Each push-up/tilt equals one repetition. Repeat 12-15 reps with 20 seconds rest.

IMPROVES BALANCE, PADDLE STRENGTH AND CORE STRENGTH

ADVANCING THE EXERCISE
You can advance this exercise further by lifting one leg during the movement.

2 V-SIT WITH COUNTER ROTATION

The goal of this exercise is to challenge your abdominal and lower back muscles as they work to stabilise this balance position. This exercise can improve torso movements during surfing. If you're an advanced surfer or a competing surfer, then this exercise on the BOSU can be invaluable in gaining additional strength.

THE START POSITION
Sit up with your hips positioned directly on top of the dome. Lean back slightly, then lift one leg at a time until the body is in a bent knee v-sit position. Hands may be placed on the sides of the dome, or may be lifted for more balance challenge. Holding the v-sit position, slowly lower your knees to one side while rotating your torso in the opposite direction. The rotation of your torso should counter balance the movement of your legs.

Return to the start position and alternate sides. Keep the movement slow and controlled. Don't allow the lower back to become rounded at any time during the exercise.

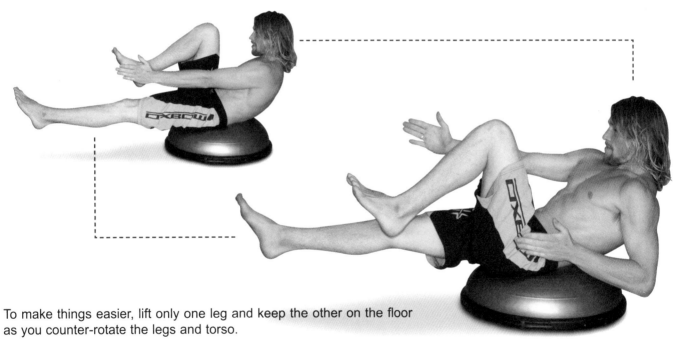

To make things easier, lift only one leg and keep the other on the floor as you counter-rotate the legs and torso.

IMPROVES BALANCE, PADDLE STRENGTH AND CORE STRENGTH

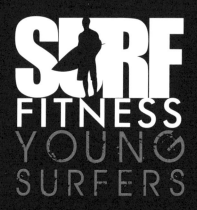

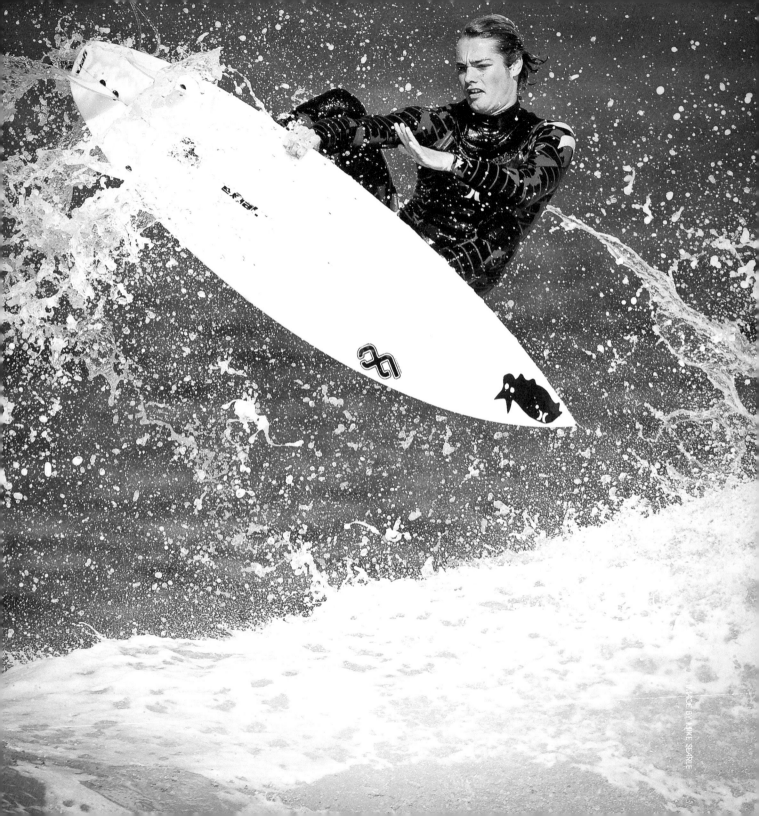

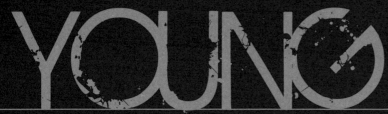

YOUNG SURFERS

LAND TRAINING FOR YOUNG SURFERS

GETTING STARTED

There are many different types of training available to young surfers. If implemented properly they can easily help you to improve your surfing and increase your fitness.

STRENGTH TRAINING can come in many different forms for young surfers. Resistance bands and exercises using your own body weight, like press-ups can be done just about anywhere. Resistance bands can help you improve your paddle power and upper body strength if supervised correctly.

CARDIOVASCULAR fitness can be boosted by swimming, which will also improve your upper body strength. If you are not a good swimmer then now is the time to improve. Any improvements made in swimming as a young surfer will be of great benefit in later life.

CORE STRENGTH exercises can be done on a weekly basis and will aid you as a young developing surfer by increasing your strength and skill levels.

WEIGHT TRAINING should be undertaken with the advice of a professional. Don't start lifting weights at too young an age. Stick to light resistance training. Low weight and high reps will improve your strength as well as your muscular endurance. Leave the weight lifting until you reach around 17-18 years of age. Until then stick to resistance bands and own body weight exercises like press-ups and pull-ups.

TOP TIPS
IMPROVING YOUR FITNESS

- Start off slowly and as your strength increases, increase your speed.

- Maintain control and good posture throughout the exercise.

- Work hard on precision and not so much on speed.

QUALITY NOT QUANTITY!

BASIC GUIDELINES FOR THE YOUNG SURFER'S FITNESS

As with all workouts, whatever your age, it's really important to follow a good warm-up procedure before any exercise and a good cool-down regime after.

8 STEPS TO IMPROVING YOUR FITNESS AND SURFING

1 IMPROVE YOUR GENERAL AEROBIC FITNESS
Great ways to do this are by swimming, running, or both!

2 IMPROVE YOUR CORE STRENGTH
Aim for at least 2 sessions a week of at least 20-30 minutes.

3 IMPROVE YOUR BALANCE
Equipment like wobble and Indo boards can be great for improving balance, co-ordination and core strength.

4 IMPROVE YOUR STRENGTH
Incorporate a resistance band section into your workouts. Make sure you get some safety advice from a professional first.

5 IMPROVE YOUR FLEXIBILITY
Adopt a positive flexibility and mobility attitude. Keeping young joints healthy and free from injury could give you that extra edge in the future.

6 TAKE YOUR CORE STRENGTH TO THE NEXT LEVEL
Introduce a medicine ball and or a Swiss ball to your core strength workout for additional core strength training. Use a lightweight medicine ball.

7 PLYOMETRIC TRAINING DRILLS
Done in a safe and controlled environment with adult supervision, plyometric training drills will aid you as a young surfer by increasing your explosive power. Be sure to follow the guidelines for warming up.

8 ADOPT A HEALTHY LIFESTYLE
A good nutritional intake will give you the energy you need to take your surfing to the next level.

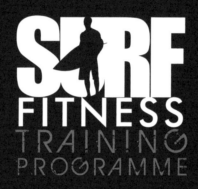

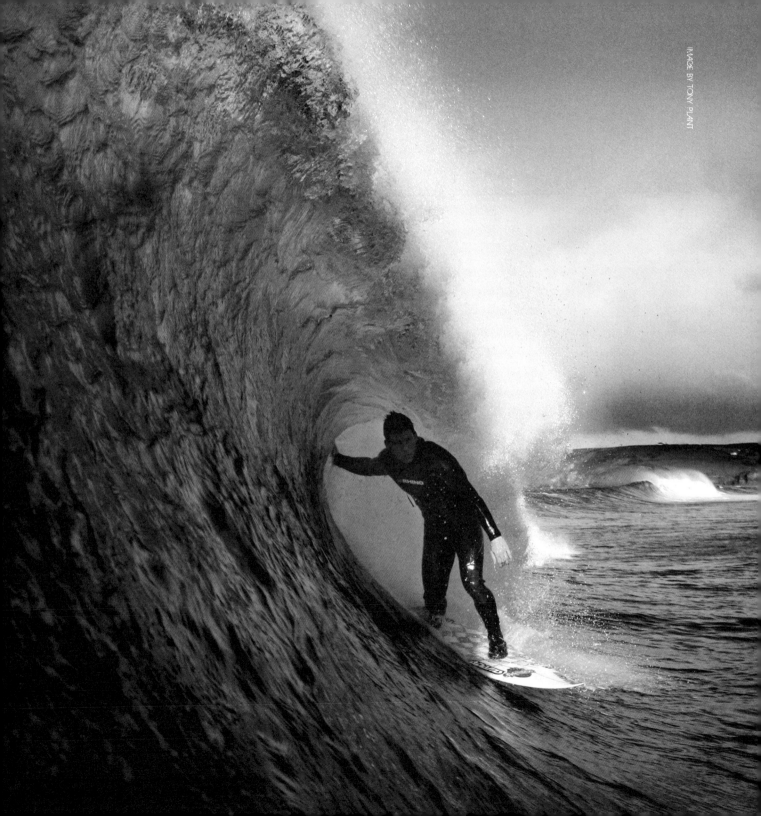

TRAINING
PROGRAMME

DESIGNING A TRAINING PROGRAMME FOR TOTAL SURF FITNESS
THE IMPORTANCE OF TAILORING A TRAINING PROGRAMME

A well-tailored land training programme will help you achieve your peak fitness goals. A good programme of work each week will allow you to maintain good progressive training principles, allowing you to surf stronger with more energy and flair. A training programme will help you prepare for your goal whether it's more paddle power, explosive speed, or just improved surfing movements.

Charting your progress each week will help you stay focused on your goals, boosting your motivation and allowing you to see your progression. The sample programmes in this section are straightforward and basic allowing you to record your performance each week.

As with any training programme a good constructive warm-up is vital; this combined with a good cool-off section will allow you to stay injury free.

The key to a good well-balanced land-based surf training programme is to tailor the programme to suit your fitness ability. Aim for exercises and movements that will strengthen your own surfing style. You may be new to surfing: a longboarder or a shortboarder looking for more strength in that new move you are just perfecting. A good selection of balance transfer exercises will allow more power through an improved range of movement.

In general, well-balanced training should contain some form of aerobic training like running or swimming. There should be some form of upper body strength training i.e. weights, resistance bands etc.

IMPORTANT
Don't just focus on your upper body and general fitness. Your legs play a vital role in surfing, keeping them injury free is a must. Focus on leg work that will keep your knees, ankles and hips strong.

TAILORING YOUR TRAINING PROGRAMME

Remember, each training section in this book is included to make you aware of the range of training types available. Each training section is different from the next and each plays a role in total surfing fitness. You may wish to pursue one and not the other; you may wish to train once a week or four times a week. It's all down to you and what you want to achieve.

A well-balanced surfing programme should build strength, improve muscle power, burn fat and keep you trim while improving your aerobic performance, improve your balance and keep you injury free!

Any well balanced flexibility programme should cover all major muscle groups and should be tailored to improve your surfing performance.

ALTERNATE AND LIMIT YOUR TRAINING TYPES

If you're training 3-4 times a week it will be beneficial to limit your sessions to 1 or 2 different training types and alternate them regularly.

MONDAY
Plyometrics and Balance Training

TUESDAY
Aerobic Training - Swim or Run

THURSDAY
Free Weights and Resistance Bands

FRIDAY
Core Strength Training and Aerobic Training

A change of training type is often better than over-training. You may wish to develop additional strength using weights during the flat season and only use resistance bands for strength when the waves are good.

TOP TIP

CHANGE YOUR TRAINING PROGRAMME REGULARLY

Changing a training programme every 8 weeks or so will allow your body to stay challenged. Mix things up to keep the body guessing.

TRAINING PROGRAMME

EXAMPLES OF SURF TRAINING PROGRAMMES

This basic programme can be changed to suit your requirements. There are many different ways to train for surfing using the training aids shown to you in this book. Remember a well-balanced training plan each week covering all major muscle groups will allow you to progress faster.

ALL OVER BODY STRENGTH TRAINING
Multi-training kit session – Gym-based or at home.

EXERCISE	SETS	REPS	REST
WARM UP 5-7 minutes of light mobility exercises and a light run			
SWISS BALL PRESS-UPS	3	6-12	30sec
BASIC LUNGE – Try static or walking lunges	3-4	6-12	30sec
SWISS BALL SHOULDER PRESS	3	6-12	20sec
TRICEPS EXTENSION – Free weights	3	6-12	20sec
FRONT RAISES/SIDE RAISES – Free weights	3	6-12	30sec
BASIC SQUATS	3	6-12	60sec
FRONT PLANK	ALAP	ALAP	ALAP
SIDE PLANK	ALAP	ALAP	ALAP
PLYOMETRIC PRESS-UPS - On floor	3-4	TSYF	TSYF
CHEST PRESS FLYES – On Swiss ball	3	6-12	30sec
PRONE MEDICINE BALL PULL OVER - Using Swiss ball	3	6-12	30sec
PLYOMETRIC UPRIGHT JUMPS	3	6-12	TSYF
REVERSE FLYES – free weights	3	6-12	TSYF
BASIC SWISS BALL CRUNCH	4-5	10-15	TSYF
COOL DOWN STRETCHING 8-10 minutes			

ALAP
As Long As Possible

TSYF
To Suit Your Fitness

SUPER SET PROGRAMME

If you get your fitness up to a good level you may wish to try advanced programming that involves super setting your exercises, taking your fitness to even greater heights! A super set workout and training plan can be very high impact but the benefits long term can be great if you are looking for supreme surfing fitness.

If you're a big-wave rider or are looking for total surfing fitness at all levels, then super setting your workout to advanced levels is a must!

Many movements will be high impact and possibly dynamic so warming up before is very important. Super sets often involve working the body to exhaustion with one exercise followed by another and sometimes as many as 4-5 exercises one after the other.

Change your super set exercise programme to suit your requirements – there is no set rule on the type of super set training you do.

WHICHEVER PROGRAMME ROUTE YOU TAKE ALWAYS WARM UP, COOL DOWN, PROGRESS AND TRY TO KEEP YOUR PROGRAMME WELL BALANCED COVERING ALL MAJOR MUSCLE GROUPS.

TRAINING PROGRAMME

SUPER SET PROGRAMME EXAMPLE

The super set programme below is for advanced levels of fitness. Before undertaking a super set training programme you should have reached a high level of fitness. Any super set programme should raise the HR to anaerobic and high aerobic levels.

SUPER SET PROGRAMME EXAMPLE

MOBILITY EXERCISES 4-5 minutes – Rest 90 seconds

BIG WARM UP 12-15 minute slow run – Rest 90 seconds

EXERCISE SEQUENCE

SET 1 Repeat twice with 90 second recovery intervals

10 x Press-Ups
10 x Plyometric Jumps – Standing
10 x Reverse Flyes
10 x Plyometric Press-Ups

SET 2 Repeat three times with 90 second recovery intervals

10 x Shoulder Press on Swiss Ball
10 x Front Side Raises Using Resistance Bands
10 x Box Jump

SET 3 Repeat four times with 90 second intervals

10 x Bench Dips
10 x Press-Ups – either normal or plyometric
10 x Triceps Extension

JUST REMEMBER TO OVERLOAD THE BODY ON EACH SET AND TAKE QUALITY REST BETWEEN SETS

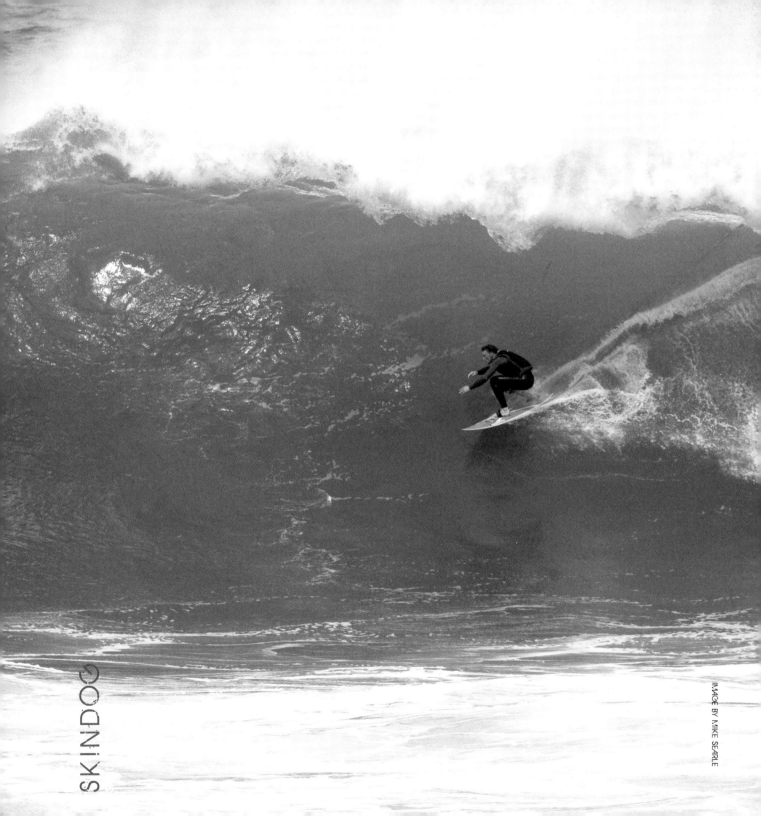

SKINDOG

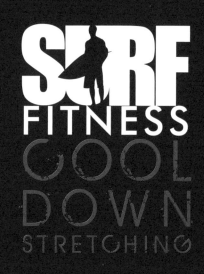

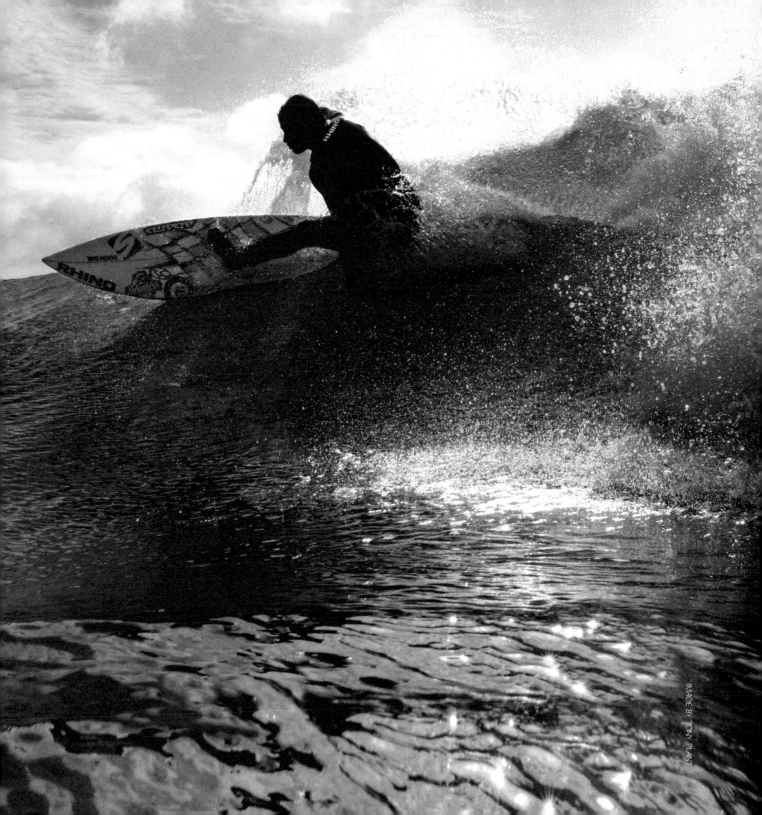

COOL-DOWN

STRETCHING

COOL-DOWN
DEVELOPMENTAL STRETCHES

POST-WORKOUT OR POST-SURF

Cooling down and stretching properly after a workout will be of great benefit to any sportsman. Slowly and gradually reducing your exercise intensity over the last 10 minutes of your session will comfortably bring your body back down to a near resting state.

As mentioned in the Introduction To Flexibility section, stretching fully is most productive after a surf or workout. Developing a basic knowledge of cool-down stretching and developmental stretching can be of great use to any surfer.

The stretches in this section will help prepare your muscles for development stretching by reducing muscular tightness.

With any stretches it is important to use slow and controlled movements taking care not to bounce or rock whilst performing the stretch. Tension should decrease as you hold the stretch, if it does not then ease off slightly and find a position that is more comfortable.

When undertaking any flexibility programme maintaining a stable body position is an important factor. Unstable body positions can cause an athlete to wobble, and this could lead to an over-stretch, muscle pull or spraining of joints.

STATIC STRETCHES

Implementing basic static stretching methods will result in less muscle soreness post surf or workout. They also have a smaller risk of possible damage to connective tissues than prolonged ballistic methods. Static stretches can be done almost anywhere and are the simplest type of stretches available to you.

DEVELOPMENTAL STRETCHING

Developmental stretching takes your flexibility to the next level. These can be held for a much longer period, between 15-30 seconds.

The developmental stretch will fine- tune your muscle and help increase your flexibility.

PNF Proprioceptive Neuromuscular Facilitation

If you want to gain super flexibility with your stretching then the PNF technique is possibly the most appropriate, however this type of exercise is not suitable for all due to it being an advanced level of stretching.

PNF involves the use of muscle contraction before the stretch in an attempt to achieve the maximum muscle stretch. In order to undertake PNF stretching effectively you will need the help of a knowledgeable training partner, experienced coach or trainer. Great care should be taken with this form of flexibility training.

When devising a well-balanced developmental flexibility programme for surfing, it is important to take into account the movements of the body while surfing. It would be beneficial as a surfer to develop a specific flexibility programme for those joints involved in the movements of surfing at all levels.

You can make effective gains in your flexibility on your own with a basic understanding of static stretching. Holding a developmental static stretch for 30 seconds or more will aid in developing your flexibility and help to take your flexibility to the next level, as opposed to cool-down stretching which will aid you with your recovery.

WITH ALL STRETCHES YOU SHOULD STICK TO THESE BASIC RULES

- Warm up your core body temperature before a surf or workout.

- Use basic mobility to start and integrate this into your light aerobic warm-up.

- Very light stretching can be done at the start of your session, but still use mobility and aerobic warm-up.

- Hold development stretches for 30 seconds or more for gains in flexibility.

- Try to seek advice on flexibility programmes and adopt a good cool-down flexibility section into your workouts or post-surf session.

STRETCHING FULLY IS MOST PRODUCTIVE AFTER A SURF OR WORK OUT

Developing a basic knowledge of cool-down stretching and developmental stretching can be of great use to any surfer.

COOL DOWN STRETCHING

1 ADDUCTOR STRETCH

This stretch is directed purely at stretching out your adductors. Stretching this area well after any exercise is important especially if you are going to be back in the surf the next day.

THE START POSITION

Sitting on the floor, bring the soles of the feet together in front of you. Gently take hold of your feet and press your knees down using your elbows until you feel a comfortable stretch in the inner thighs. Take care to keep the back straight during the stretch.

It's important you don't over-stretch during this exercise. If it hurts at any point ease back the pressure on your knees slightly until you are comfortable

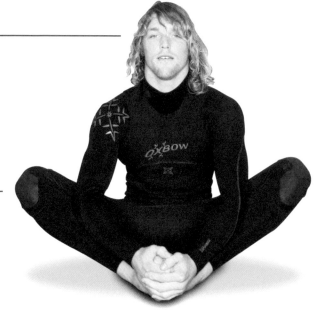

Hold the stretch for 15-20 seconds.

AIDS INJURY PREVENTION

2 SEATED LAT STRETCH

This stretch will stretch your obliques and latissimus dorsi, both of which are important for paddling.

THE START POSITION

Sitting on the floor, cross your legs and place one hand on the floor out to the side. Extend your other arm directly above your head and reach over past your opposite shoulder.

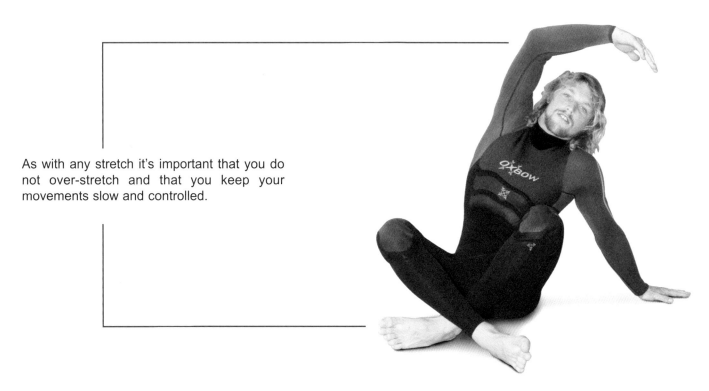

As with any stretch it's important that you do not over-stretch and that you keep your movements slow and controlled.

Hold for 15-20 seconds and repeat on the opposite side.

AIDS INJURY PREVENTION

3 STANDING DELTOID STRETCH
This will stretch out your deltoids.

THE START POSITION
Start by standing with your feet hip width apart. Slowly take your right arm across your chest and gently press down on the back of your arm, avoiding any pressure on the joints. You should feel a slight stretch in your right shoulder.

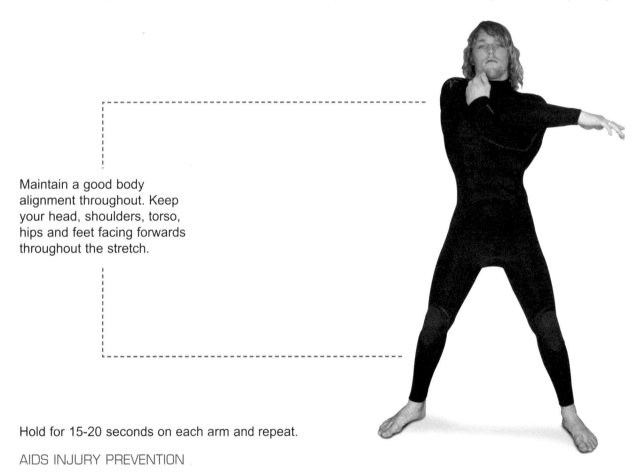

Maintain a good body alignment throughout. Keep your head, shoulders, torso, hips and feet facing forwards throughout the stretch.

Hold for 15-20 seconds on each arm and repeat.

AIDS INJURY PREVENTION

4 STANDING TRICEPS STRETCH
This will specifically stretch out your triceps.

THE START POSITION
Start by standing with your feet hip width apart, place your left hand behind your shoulder blades and with your right hand on the elbow, gently press your left arm downwards by pressing down slowly.

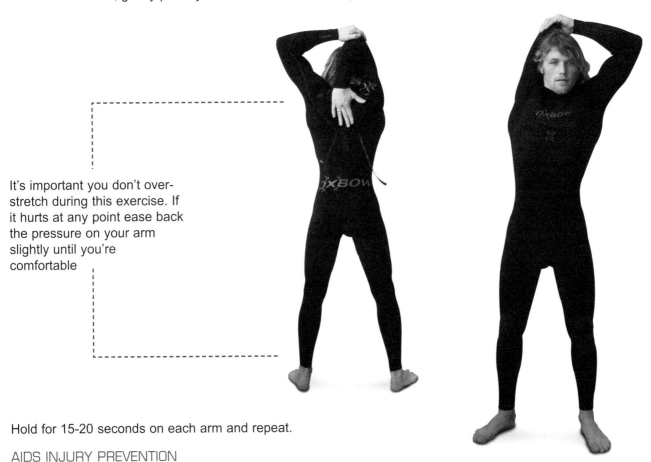

It's important you don't over-stretch during this exercise. If it hurts at any point ease back the pressure on your arm slightly until you're comfortable

Hold for 15-20 seconds on each arm and repeat.

AIDS INJURY PREVENTION

5 SEATED HAMSTRING STRETCH
This stretch will isolate your hamstrings.

THE START POSITION

Start by sitting on the floor. Straighten your left leg with your toes pointing upwards. Slightly bend your right leg bringing your heel back towards you, holding it in a comfortable position.

Slowly reach forward running your hands down the length of your extended leg until you feel a comfortable stretch in the hamstring of your left leg.

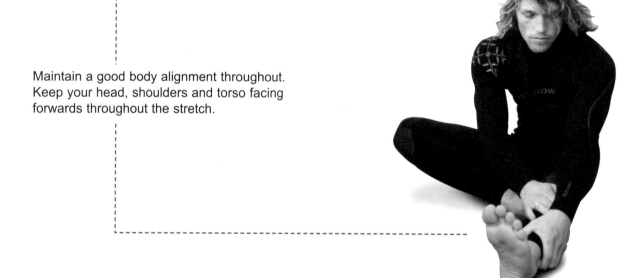

Maintain a good body alignment throughout. Keep your head, shoulders and torso facing forwards throughout the stretch.

Hold for 15-20 seconds and then repeat the stretch on your opposite leg.

AIDS INJURY PREVENTION

6 CHEST AND SHOULDER STRETCH

Stretches out pectorals and major and anterior deltoids.

THE START POSITION

Sit on the floor with your legs crossed in front of you. Place both hands flat on the floor behind your back with your hands facing backwards.

Slowly push your chest upwards and extend it out until you feel a comfortable stretch across your chest.

It's important you don't overstretch during this exercise. If you feel uncomfortable reduce the intensity of the stretch

Hold for 15-20 seconds and repeat.

AIDS INJURY PREVENTION

7 ERECTOR SPINE STRETCH
Specifically targets your erector spine (the muscles that support the spine).

THE START POSITION
Start by kneeling on a flat surface on all fours. Place your hands flat on the floor directly under your shoulders.

Gently pull your tummy in and slowly round your spine. Hold this position to feel the stretch.

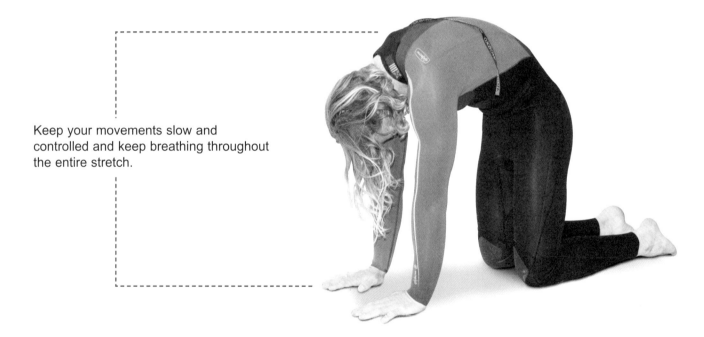

Keep your movements slow and controlled and keep breathing throughout the entire stretch.

Hold for 15-20 seconds.

AIDS INJURY PREVENTION

8 OUTER HIP STRETCH

This will stretch your hip abductors.

THE START POSITION

Start by sitting with your right leg flat on the floor straight out in front of you and your left leg across it.

Use the forearm of your right arm to gently push down on the outside of your left knee, slowly easing the bent leg across the chest and in towards it.

It's important you don't over-stretch during this exercise. If you feel uncomfortable reduce the intensity of the stretch

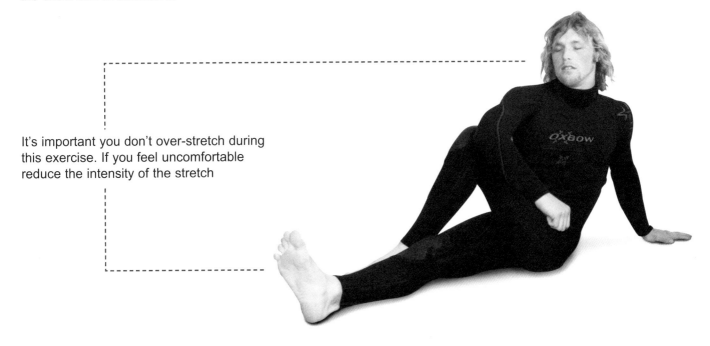

You should feel a stretch on the outer hip. If it hurts at any point ease off until you feel more comfortable.

Hold for 15-20 seconds and repeat on the opposite leg.

AIDS INJURY PREVENTION

9 INNER THIGH STRETCH
This will stretch out your adductors.

THE START POSITION
Step forwards onto your left foot, place your hands on your left leg and keeping your back straight and your head up bend your left leg to a 90^0 angle. Keep your shoulders over your pelvis throughout the stretch. You should feel a comfortable stretch in the inner thigh of your right leg.

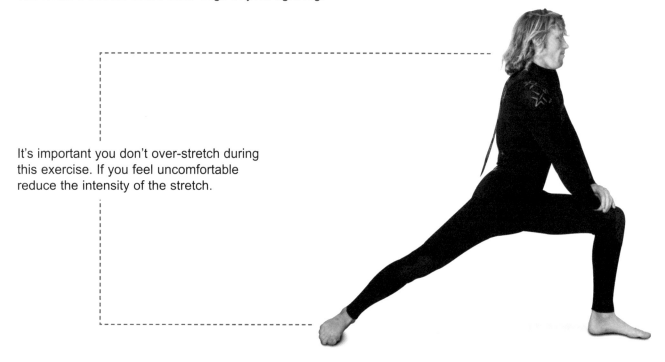

It's important you don't over-stretch during this exercise. If you feel uncomfortable reduce the intensity of the stretch.

Care should be taken not to bend forwards and you should keep your right foot turned outwards to avoid any strain on the knee.

Hold for 15-20 seconds and repeat on your opposite leg.

AIDS INJURY PREVENTION

10 STANDING QUADRICEPS STRETCH
This will specifically target your quadriceps.

THE START POSITION
Bend your left leg and slowly draw your heel towards your bottom. Keep the back straight with knees together and hips facing forwards. Initially you may wish to use a wall or another solid object for support.

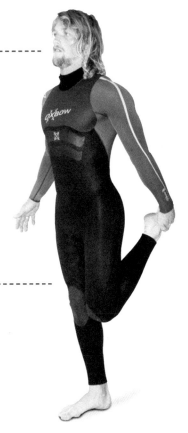

It's important you don't over-stretch during this exercise. If you feel uncomfortable reduce the intensity of the stretch.

Only pull your heel up as far as is comfortable and if you feel any pain during the stretch ease off slightly.

Hold for 15-20 seconds and repeat on your opposite leg.

AIDS INJURY PREVENTION

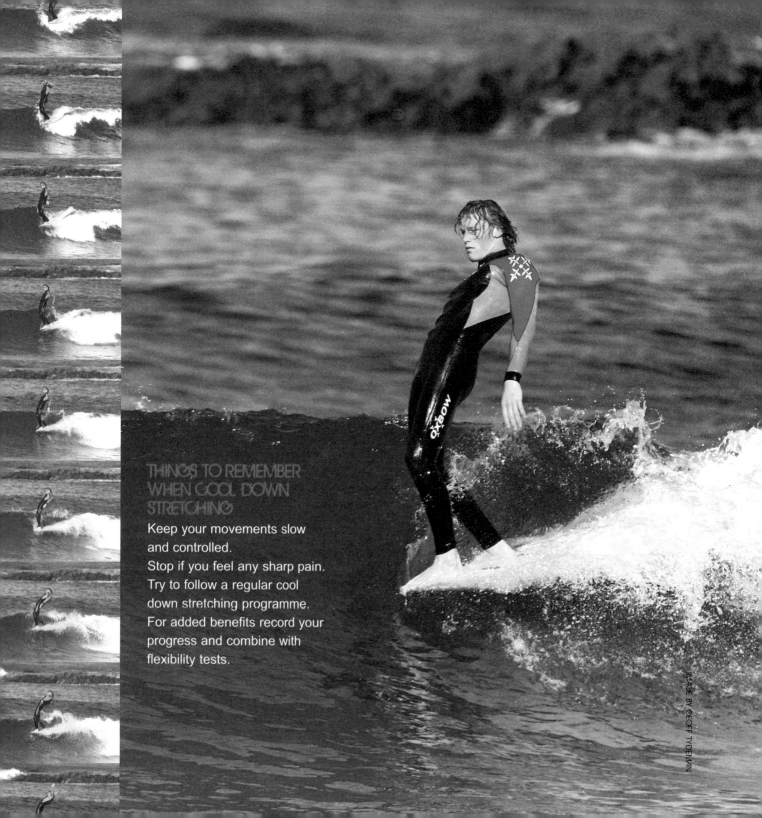

THINGS TO REMEMBER WHEN COOL DOWN STRETCHING

Keep your movements slow and controlled.
Stop if you feel any sharp pain.
Try to follow a regular cool down stretching programme.
For added benefits record your progress and combine with flexibility tests.

11 STANDING CALF STRETCH

This will stretch your gastrocnemius.

THE START POSITION

Start by positioning your left foot behind you and slightly bending your right knee. Keep your left leg straight and slowly press down your heel towards the floor until you feel the stretch in your calf muscle.

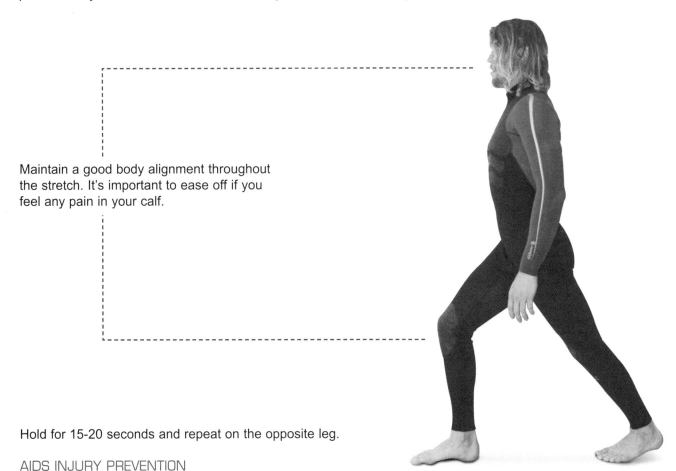

Maintain a good body alignment throughout the stretch. It's important to ease off if you feel any pain in your calf.

Hold for 15-20 seconds and repeat on the opposite leg.

AIDS INJURY PREVENTION

12 ABDOMINAL STRETCH
This stretch specifically targets your rectus abdominus.

THE START POSITION
Start by lying on the floor with your hands either side of your chest in a press-up position. Keep your hips on the floor and slowly push up lifting through your chest, gently arching your back.

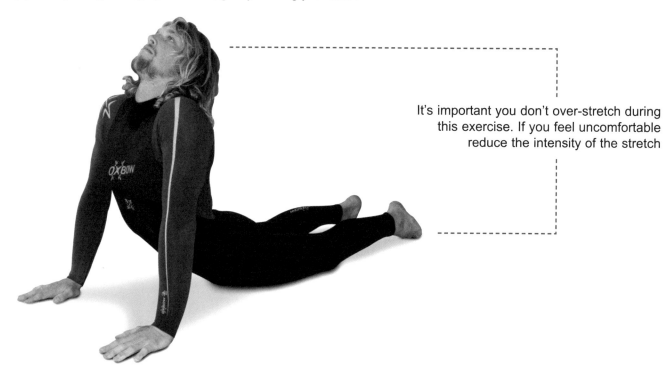

It's important you don't over-stretch during this exercise. If you feel uncomfortable reduce the intensity of the stretch

Take care to maintain a slow and controlled movement throughout the stretch.

Hold for 15-20 seconds.

AIDS INJURY PREVENTION

13 LYING GLUTEAL STRETCH
Stretches your erector spine

THE START POSITION
Start by lying on your back on the floor with your legs out straight. Leaving your left leg out straight, bend your right leg slowly flexing your right knee and pull it upwards and across your body towards your left shoulder.

Keep your shoulders flat on the floor throughout the stretch. Extending your right arm out to the side keeping it flat on the floor will help you to do this.

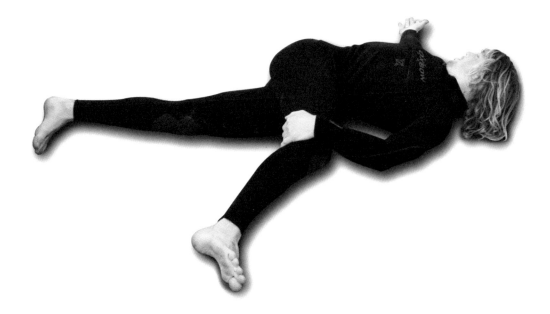

Make sure you have plenty of space for this stretch and keep your movements slow and controlled.

Hold for 15-20 seconds.

AIDS INJURY PREVENTION

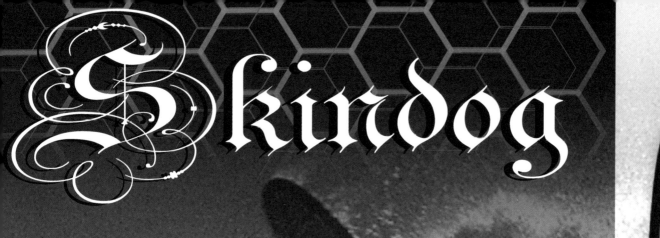

Skindog

Featured model: 9'0" CRT AR

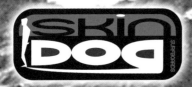

High performance longboards by Ben skinner

1 SWISS BALL COOL DOWN STRETCHES - SHOULDER STRETCH
This stretch will stretch out your deltoids.

THE START POSITION
Kneel on the floor close to the ball, with your upper arm resting on top of it. Keeping your head up, lower your body toward the ball. As you do this you should feel a stretch along the back of your shoulder.

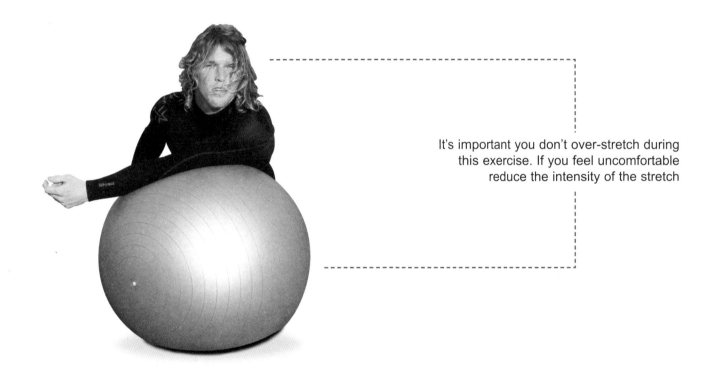

It's important you don't over-stretch during this exercise. If you feel uncomfortable reduce the intensity of the stretch

Hold for 20-30 seconds and then repeat on the opposite arm. Repeat on both arms 3-4 times.

AIDS INJURY PREVENTION

COOL DOWN STRETCHING

2 STANDING HIP FLEXOR STRETCH
This will stretch your hip flexor.

THE START POSITION
Start by standing with the top of your right foot placed on the ball and your left foot flat on the floor. Slowly lower your body bending your left leg. You should feel a mild stretch on the inside right leg.

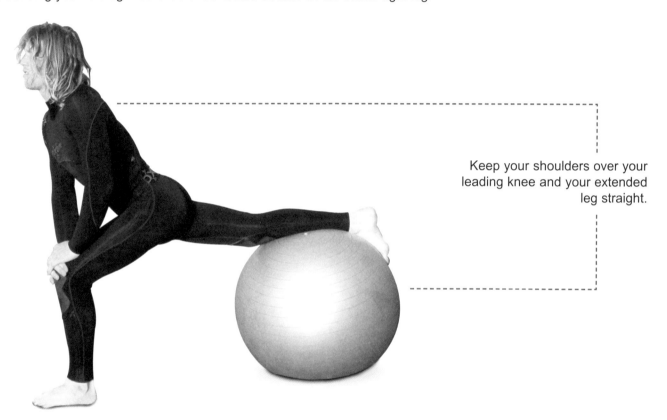

Keep your shoulders over your leading knee and your extended leg straight.

Hold for 20-30 seconds on each leg. Repeat on both legs 3-4 times.

AIDS INJURY PREVENTION

3 LATERAL STRETCH

This stretch specifically targets your latissimus dorsi.

THE START POSITION

Start by kneeling on the floor with one hand on top of the ball at arm's length. Keep your head down and sit back on your heels. Lower your shoulder towards the floor until you feel a mild stretch along the side of your back.

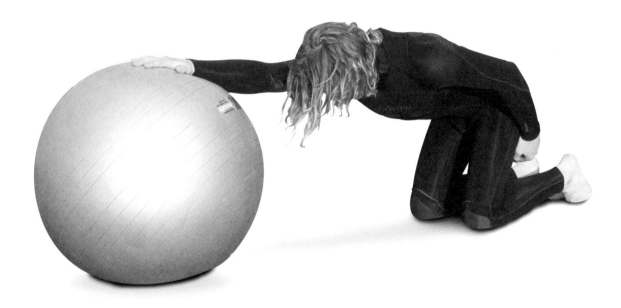

Hold for 20-30 seconds on each arm. Repeat on both arms 3-4 times.

AIDS INJURY PREVENTION

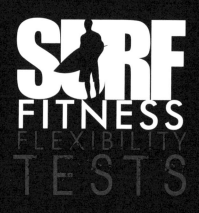

SURF FITNESS

FLEXIBILITY

TESTS

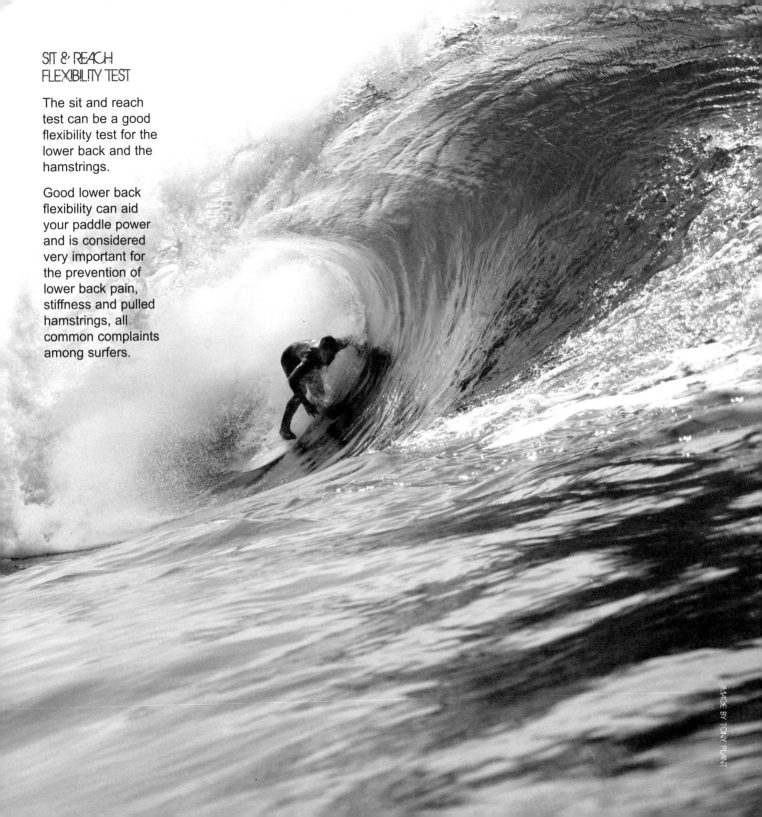

SIT & REACH FLEXIBILITY TEST

The sit and reach test can be a good flexibility test for the lower back and the hamstrings.

Good lower back flexibility can aid your paddle power and is considered very important for the prevention of lower back pain, stiffness and pulled hamstrings, all common complaints among surfers.

FLEXIBILITY TESTS

PERFORMING A SIT AND REACH TEST

This is a very simple test but is an excellent way of charting the increase in your flexibility.

GUIDELINES FOR SIT AND REACH TEST

Sit on the floor with your legs out straight and your shoes off. Place the soles of your feet against a flat surface that you can place a ruler or tape measure on the top of. You can use anything from an exercise step to a coffee table for this as long as it's low enough and won't move during the test. With your legs perfectly straight, bend forward at the hips using your lower back muscles and try to touch your toes.

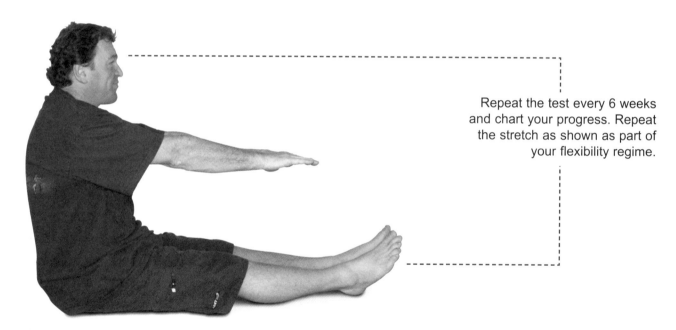

Repeat the test every 6 weeks and chart your progress. Repeat the stretch as shown as part of your flexibility regime.

If you can, reach past your toes and place your hands on the box. Repeat this 3 times and record either how far your fingers are from your toes or how far past your toes you can reach using the ruler.

THE AIM OF THE SIT AND REACH TEST IS TO HIGHLIGHT TIGHTNESS IN THE LOWER BACK AND HAMSTRING MUSCLES

TO ASSESS YOUR PERFORMANCE PLEASE USE THE CHART BELOW

FLEXIBILITY RATING	MEN (CM FROM TOES)	WOMEN (CM FROM TOES)
EXCELLENT	BETWEEN 17 AND 27	BETWEEN 21 AND 30
GOOD	BETWEEN 6 AND 16	BETWEEN 11 AND 20
AVERAGE	BETWEEN 0 AND 5	BETWEEN 1 AND 10
FAIR	BETWEEN -8 AND -1	BETWEEN -7 AND 0
POOR	BETWEEN -19 AND -9	BETWEEN -14 AND -8
VERY POOR	-20 AND BELOW	-15 AND BELOW

If you want to improve your score it's a good idea to stretch the hamstrings out at least 3 times a week and incorporate the stretch in to your full body flexibility programme.

EXAMPLE OF A SIMPLE FLEXIBILITY CHART TO BE COMPLETED EACH SESSION
Keeping a record of your progress will help you to isolate areas that may need more attention.

MUSCLES STRETCHED	DURATION	NO OF SETS	STIFFNESS
ADDUCTORS	30 SECONDS	3 SETS	NONE

If you can spare the time several flexibility sessions a week can be a major boost to your overall surfing fitness. Once flexibility becomes part of your regular training and surfing routine you will soon start to feel the benefits. If you are finding stretching sessions tiresome or boring then partner stretches may be of use but – seek advice from a professional before stretching to the limit!

FLEXIBILITY TESTS

TRUNK EXTENSION TEST

In addition to the Sit and Reach Test, a Trunk Extension Test may be of some benefit. This basic test allows the surfer to evaluate the amount of backward bend (extension) possible in the spine.

The procedure is simple, however take care. This is a movement that should be pain free and done very slowly. If you do suffer from any lower back injuries then this exercise should be avoided.

PERFORMING A TRUNK EXTENSION TEST

GUIDELINES FOR TRUNK EXTENSION TEST

* Start by lying face down with your hands palms down by your shoulders and your elbows drawn in by your sides.

* Next slowly raise the front of your upper body off the floor attempting to keep the hip bone in contact with the floor.

* Make sure that the movement is not forced in any way and that you stop when the hip bones start to come off the floor.

* Evaluate trunk extension using the table below.

EVALUATION OF TRUNK FLEXIBILITY

EXTENSION	CHARACTERISTICS
GOOD	Your hips should remain in contact with the floor while your arms are fully extended
FAIR	The hip bones lift off the floor up to two inches
POOR	The hip bones lift off the floor two inches or more

The lower back area takes a certain amount of strain during paddling, and a good strong core and abdominal area can help boost the strength of the lower back. In addition to core strength training, a good back stretching routine can be of great benefit to the overall flexibility of the trunk.

HIP FLEXION – HAMSTRING FLEXIBILITY

There are ways available to test a surfer's flexibility. The Hip Flexion – Hamstring Flexibility Test evaluates the range of motion in the hips and tightness of the hamstrings. This is an area that many surfers have a problem with due to the nature of many surfing movements.

HIP FLEXION – HAMSTRING FLEXIBILITY TEST

GUIDELINES FOR TEST

- Start by lying flat on your back.

- Hold left leg down with your right hand to stabilise the pelvis and use your left hand to passively raise your right leg.

- Ensure that you keep the leg straight and only go as far as is comfortable.

- See chart below to evaluate your hip flexibility.

EVALUATION OF HIP FLEXIBILITY

EXTENSION	CHARACTERISTICS
90%	Your leg is raised beyond a 90 degree angle while your pelvis remains in a neutral position.
POOR	Your leg is raised to an angle of 80-90 degrees with the pelvis in a neutral position.
FAIR	Your leg is raised less than 80 degrees without the knee bending or the alignment of the pelvis being compromised.

Tightness of the hamstrings can place undue stress on the lower back; this can increase the risk of injury.

THESE ARE JUST A FEW OF THE TESTS YOU CAN USE TO TEST FLEXIBILITY. REMEMBER THAT A GOOD FLEXIBILITY PROGRAMME FOR ANY SURFER CAN AID INJURY PREVENTION.

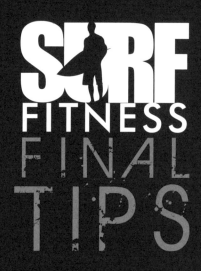

SURF FITNESS
FINAL TIPS

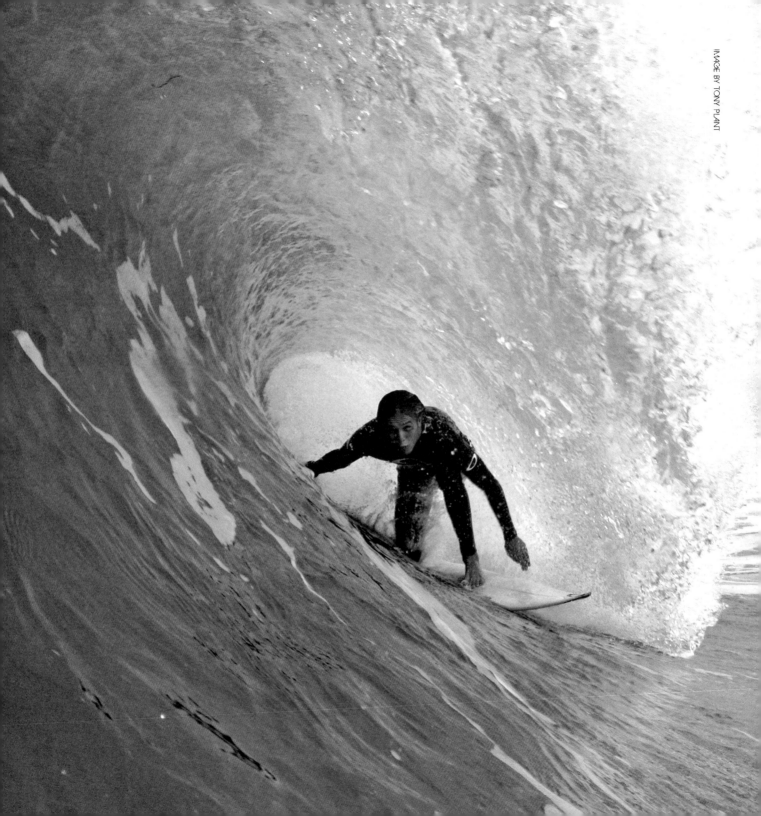

INJURY PREVENTION

A FEW EXTRA TIPS ON INJURY PREVENTION

- Try to avoid any training when you're tired.

- Maintain a good, healthy diet.

- Don't overdo it! Ease your way into any new training programme with care and build exercises up slowly as your strength and fitness improve.

- If you experience any pain during a training session or a surf, no matter how good the waves are, STOP! Your body is trying to tell you something.

- When doing any high-impact exercises like plyometrics, use correct surfaces that won't damage joints.

- Try to allow plenty of time for warming up and cooling down!

- If you run try to avoid roads and pavements. Try a softer surface like grass.

- Visiting a good sports massage therapist can be of great benefit. They can aid recovery and guide you in the right direction when it comes to preventing further injuries.

- A good flexibility programme can be worth its weight in gold. It's worth the effort so adopt one today!

- Use correct training shoes. A good sound running trainer is essential. Iinjuries like runner's knee may occur from running in incorrect shoes. In addition to runner's knee you may be at risk from stress fractures that can be caused from over-training or doing too much too soon!

THE GOLDEN RULE TO INJURY PREVENTION IS TO USE YOUR COMMON SENSE

If it hurts, stop – prevention is better than cure. Don't expect to go from zero to hero overnight but remember with a little hard work you'll soon be reaping the benefits and charging harder and faster than ever.

SURFING INJURIES

If you're unlucky enough to get an injury while surfing or exercising then take action. Don't just shrug it off and think it will go away.

If you've twisted a knee, ankle, elbow, etc then follow the RICE procedure! RICE is the simplest and most effective remedy for a whole range of possible surfing injuries.

The procedure of Rest, Ice, Compression and Elevation will help reduce swelling and can help slow down the bruising effect of an injury. Both of these can often slow down the healing process!

As soon as possible after you get an injury, you should try to apply ice and raise the injured limb.

Very often it is the first few hours that are the most important in getting some treatment. If you can, rest the injured part for at least 48 hours!

While using ice to aid the healing process try to apply it for around 10 minutes every hour. This can reduce any bleeding from torn blood vessels. A makeshift ice pack can be put together using a tea towel or cloth.

To help control any swelling, bandage the injured area firmly but not too tightly. If the bandage becomes too loose, tighten it accordingly.

Elevation will allow blood flow towards the heart and this will reduce pressure on the injured area.

RICE IS ONLY A SORT TERM MEASURE. IF YOU SUSPECT A SERIOUS INJURY SEEK A PROFESSIONAL'S ADVICE!

It's important that you give yourself enough time to recover from an injury. If you go back to exercise before you are ready you could do permanent damage.

FINAL TIPS

FUELLING YOUR SURF SESSION

Any good sportsman knows the value of a well-balanced diet. If you're lucky enough to surf on a regular basis then a good healthy diet can make all the difference to your surfing session.

Eating a diet rich in carbohydrates can boost your energy levels allowing you to surf just that bit longer. At the same time, if you are training on a regular basis for additional gains in surf strength, then a healthy balanced diet can boost your training sessions.

Carbohydrates, proteins and indeed fats are all used by the body and provide energy for exercise; however the best form of fuel for a training or surf session can be found in complex carbohydrates like rice, pasta and potatoes.

Eat plenty of vegetables! Eating bright green vegetables in particular as part of a balanced diet will boost your energy levels. Starting your day with slow-release energy foods like muesli, oats and maltose bread is a great way to fuel a dawny surf session and will give you a great base for the day ahead.

FUELLING YOUR RECOVERY

During a training session or surf, a sports drink is thought by many to be better than water at speeding up recovery, particularly if it has been a hot day or you are surfing for long periods during the day.

A good sports drink will contain sodium which will help towards a good electrolyte balance. Electrolytes are mineral salts (sodium, potassium and magnesium) that are dissolved in the fluids of the body. They help to regulate the fluid balance in the body like the amount of fluid in and outside the muscle cells and the amount of water in the blood stream. Your sports drink should also contain carbohydrate as this will help your body absorb water as well as giving you an energy boost.

TOP TIP

THINGS TO REMEMBER
Always stay well hydrated during the session, whether surfing or working out as good hydration will aid sporting performance.
A well-balanced carbohydrate intake will also aid your surfing session. When possible start your day with slow release carbohydrates like porridge or muesli.

EXAMPLES OF PRE SURF OR TRAINING SESSION MEALS

2-3 HOURS BEFORE TRAINING OR SURF

- Jacket potato and beans
- Pasta and sauce
- Light stir fry with noodles
- Porridge or wholegrain cereal
- Light tuna and rice salad

1-2 HOURS BEFORE TRAINING OR SURF

Fresh fruit can be a great source of carbohydrates just before a surf or workout or a fruit smoothie can be a great source of quick-release energy in the from of fructose.

IN ADDITION TO YOUR FOOD INTAKE IT IS VERY IMPORTANT TO MAINTAIN A WELL-HYDRATED BODY DURING YOUR TRAINING SESSION.

Drinking enough water throughout the day can prepare you for a workout or surf. In addition to water there are many sports drinks on the market that can aid hydration and help maintain performance. As previously stated these may aid recovery from a surf when fluid losses are high due to the length of the session.